As a Men's Health Physiotherapist dealing with pr[...] out for my patients. Resources for 'real men' are r[...] pain and erectile dysfunction the lack of informati[...] male patients have taught me, any reduction in p[...] personal empowerment and masculinity. The sub[...] his relationships should not be underestimated. Be[...] endure!!

Dr. Susie Gronski's **Pelvic Pain: The Ultimate Cock Block** provides both answers and solutions towards regaining your manpower in a factual, yet humorous way. Covering all bases, she perfectly pitches all you need to know about male anatomy, pain science, brain training, sexual function, exercise and treatment options. Written in a language style that every man and his partner will relate to, I cannot more highly recommend this text. So if you've got a spare hour or two—be kind to yourself! You'll find there's a toolbox of skills to help regain your pride and your passion...and an end to the 'cock block' in your jocks!

Hey—it may just be the best investment you'll ever make!! PROST!

JO MILIOS, MEN'S HEALTH PHYSIOTHERAPIST, WESTERN AUSTRALIA
www.menshealthphysiotherapy.com.au

Pelvic Pain: The Ultimate Cock Block by Dr. Susie Gronski is an expertly written book on male pelvic pain conditions, including Chronic Pelvic Pain Syndrome (CPPS) and Chronic Prostatitis (CP). It is a must read for patients (and their partners) wanting to take control of their symptoms and their recovery. This honest and open guide offers a window into Susie's highly reputable approach to male pelvic pain balancing hard science, humour and very practical, easy to implement self care techniques. This beautifully illustrated upfront self help guide is THE book for patients who wish to be the driver in their recovery, not just a passenger.

KARL MONAHAN IS THE FOUNDER OF THE PELVIC PAIN CLINIC IN LONDON,
A CLINIC SOLELY DEDICATED TO THE TREATMENT OF MALE PELVIC PAIN CONDITIONS.
www.thepelvicpainclinic.co.uk

Dr. Susie Gronski, a gifted physical therapist, has written a ground-breaking book on male pelvic pain. **Pelvic Pain: The Ultimate Cock Block** is a user-friendly guide that helps men understand why they have pain and what to do about it. Male pelvic pain is a forgotten piece of our health care puzzle and Dr. Gronski brings it back to life in an easy-to-read manual that every man experiencing pelvic pain should have on their bookshelf. I really enjoyed Dr. Gronski's writing style and the exercises with illustrations presented are so easy to follow. If you're a guy suffering from pelvic pain, don't hesitate to pick up a copy and begin your journey to becoming pain-free!

DR. NIKOLAS HEDBERG, AUTHOR OF THE COMPLETE THYROID HEALTH & DIET GUIDE
www.drhedberg.com

I was a male in my late 50's in a new relationship who began experiencing an ache in what felt like the bottom of my being that intensified after sexual activity. Over about 8 months, it worsened. Neither my MD or a urologist had any specific ideas for relief, so I suffered physically and with doubts about my viability going forward until I got a newsletter from my doctor describing Dr. Susie's practice.

It would be difficult to overstate how helpful Dr. Susie was from the time I made contact with her to after only our third session, by which time the ache had largely disappeared and I was able to be sexually active without pain. I now have techniques and a way of understanding and managing so the ache is either non-existent or a relatively minor and temporary inconvenience.

I highly recommend seeing Dr. Susie for any and all male issues in the nether regions.

ANONYMOUS, USA

PELVIC PAIN
THE ULTIMATE
C⊘CK BLOCK

A no bullsh*t guide to help you
navigate through pelvic pain

DR. SUSIE GRONSKI DPT, PRPC, WCS

S_G

Cover design: bookdesignbysaso.com.au
Internal design and typesetting: bookdesignbysaso.com.au
Illustrations by Veronica Zubek at Two Easels

Dr. Susie Gronski, Inc.
135 Cherry Street
Asheville, NC 28801
drsusieg.com

Printed in the United States of America

Library of Congress Cataloging-in-Publication data
Library of Congress Control Number: 2017902608

Gronski, Susie, 1985-
Pelvic Pain The Ultimate Cock Block: A no bullsh*t guide to help you navigate through pelvic pain / Susie Gronski
p. cm.
Includes bibliographical references
ISBN 978-0-9986957-0-9 (paperback)
ISBN 978-0-9986957-1-6 (e-book)

DISCLAIMER

This information is being provided to you for educational and informational purposes only. It is being provided to educate you about *pelvic health and wellness* as a self-help tool for your own use. It is not intended *to be a substitute for professional diagnosis or treatment*. This information is to be used at your own risk, based on your own judgement. For the author's full disclaimer, please go to drsusieg.com/disclaimer.

AFFILIATE DISCLOSURE

From time to time, the author may promote, affiliate with, or partner with other individuals or businesses whose programs, products and services align with her own. The author is highly selective and only promotes partners whose programs, products and/or services she respects. In the spirit of transparency, please be aware that there may be instances when this book promotes, markets, shares or sells programs, products or services for other partners and in exchange the author may receive financial compensation or other rewards. For the author's full affiliate disclosure, please go to drsusieg.com/disclaimer.

INTERACTIVE VIDEO LIBRARY

Along with the purchase of this book, you'll receive exclusive access to a private video membership site with videos demonstrating various hands-on techniques and exercises. Please visit drsusieg.com/book to activate your membership. There are reminders throughout the book that will guide you to the video library for any needed clarification or extra resources.

DEDICATIONS

To all the men who've been told they 'just have to live with it' for the rest of their lives.

To my mom and little brother because without them I wouldn't be who I am today.

To my husband for always believing in me and encouraging me to do the impossible.

To my coach, Lisa Holland, who pushed me out of my comfort zone and discovered that my real voice needed to write this book.

And finally, to my patients for all their support and encouragement. You inspire me every day and fuel my passion for learning.

Much love and gratitude to you all!

D. Susie G.

FOREWORD

It's my great pleasure to be writing the foreword for *Pelvic Pain: The Ultimate Cock Block*. Given the up-front nature of Dr. Susie Gronski's style of writing, I also need to be up-front and inform you that I'm female and have no idea what it's like to have a penis.

But I do have an immense idea about living with chronic pelvic pain. In fact, it's been over nine years since I dropped onto a concrete floor when a fit ball that I was sitting on as my office chair suddenly burst.

Pain where you don't want pain is really difficult to deal with. As a woman, I've found that I get a hearing. (I don't mean all those hearing me actually understood me – that's another story.) Yet, men with chronic pain find it even more difficult to seek and find help.

But it appears you sought help and it's in your hands right now!

I have been contacted by many males through my blog asking where they might be able to find help. They have expressed their frustrations to me because they feel they have no-one else they can speak to.

So I wasn't going to pass up the chance to write this foreword after meeting Dr. Susie and especially after reading her brilliant resource. The information Dr. Susie shares to help manage incredibly personal chronic pain doesn't just relate to men. I could relate too. I found *Pelvic Pain: The Ultimate Cock Block* useful for my own chronic pain management. In fact, when I experience pain now, I turn up Dr. Susie's fabulous mantra: 'I'm sore but I'm safe.'

It makes me believe that I'm doing something about the pain and changing the way my brain communicates it.

Could Dr. Susie have written something for us femmes too? Of course, with her eyes shut I expect! But I really like the fact male chronic pain is solely addressed here because it's important enough to warrant 100% attention.

Pelvic Pain: The Ultimate Cock Block addresses a painful – but not as complex as you might think – male chronic pain issue. And it does so in simple, straight-up language.

Start reading, get managing. Your penis is waiting!

Soula Mantalvanos

Author of Art & Chronic Pain – A Self Portrait, advocate for pelvic chronic pain, artist and creative director, and creator of *Pain Train: my online health record*

CONTENTS

INTRODUCTION

You woke up one morning expecting a hard on, but instead all you felt was dick pain. You're thinking maybe it was a weird sex position or that sports injury from the other day. "No biggie, it'll go away," you think to yourself. Or maybe you have no clue how this happened but you were sure it would eventually go away. Now you're not so sure...

Years later, you're still dealing with the same nightmare and have no answers. Like Bill Murray in the *Groundhog Day* movie, same sh*t, different day. You've tried everything but the medications haven't worked and the doctors don't know what else to do. Your penis just doesn't work the same anymore. You think about it all the time, freaked out that there's something else more serious going on that the docs just haven't found yet.

Did I hit the nail on the head?

You're probably thinking to yourself, 'But you're a chick. What do you know about having penis pain?' And you're right. Last I checked, I don't have a penis.

To be honest, I'm simply fed up with the lack of care that guys get going to traditional medical providers. I've seen too many of you walk into my clinic complaining of pelvic pain that's been wreaking havoc in your life for years. It's not necessary.

Oftentimes, physicians are unaware or lack knowledge about persistent pelvic pain. Some are even scared to tackle these symptoms because they don't know what to do other than prescribe you antibiotics, antidepressants or pain medications. Of course, then there's all the googling that you've probably done about your condition.

Let me guess... You're feeling straight up bummed and hopeless. Like there's no cure and you're just going to have to get used to living this way. Wrong! It's not 'all in your head.' And no, you don't have to live with it for the rest of your life. Who the hell wants to live like that?

You've got to know all your options and become the expert in your own health. That's why I've written this book to help guys like you realize that pelvic pain isn't permanent, making sure you know those options, to better care for yourself and take matters 'into your own hands.' You can have your life back and I'm going to tell you how.

Okay, no more beating around the bush. Let's get to it and understand what persistent pelvic pain is all about and what you can do about it.

CHAPTER 1

WHAT PELVIC PAIN IS... AND WHAT IT'S NOT

PERSISTENT VERSUS CHRONIC

In the medical world, you've probably most often seen this pelvic condition labeled as 'chronic' pelvic pain syndrome (CPPS) or chronic prostatitis. Both are used frequently and highly applicable in the medical practice, but these terms are not always inclusive when it comes to having pain 'down there.'

In this book, you'll never seen me address your pain as a 'chronic' condition. Why? Well, because when I hear the word 'chronic', I think 'permanent' and that's not what your symptoms are. Changing the way you think about your pain is the first step to healing. Knowing that your symptoms are persistent but can be resolved is oh-so liberating. Those fears about maybe living with pain for the rest of your life can go away. So let's take the word 'chronic' out of your vocabulary starting right now.

SO, WHAT IS PERSISTENT PELVIC PAIN?

Male pelvic pain sits in a lot of categories and comes with a lot of tags. Sorta like a smorgasbord list of symptoms that classify if you have persistent pelvic pain or not. For the sake of consistency in what you read on the internet and in books, most male pelvic pain is classified by the government research organization National Institute of Health (NIH) as chronic prostatitis or chronic pelvic pain syndrome (CPPS).

If you want to get real technical, the NIH classifies prostatitis into four categories:

I   Acute bacterial prostatitis
II Chronic bacterial prostatitis
III Chronic non-bacterial prostatitis
    ❯ IIIA inflammatory
    ❯ IIIB non-inflammatory
IV Asymptomatic inflammatory prostatitis

Any word with '-itis' at the end of it means inflammation, so you can see how these four are related to inflammation already.

Now, 95% of persistent pelvic pain cases are Type III non-bacterial prostatitis. The most important take away message is that only 5% of cases are actually caused by an active bacterial infection. Which means the likelihood of bacteria causing the problem is low. Typically, when there's an infection present, you have symptoms of fever, chills, pain, genital pain, pain with urination, blood in urine, etc.

For true bacterial 'itis', antibiotics are totally acceptable as a treatment plan and will most likely clear things up. But if not treated right, acute bacterial prostatitis can become chronic or persistent. This occurs in only 5% of bacterial cases.

Chronic bacterial prostatitis requires a more aggressive treatment with antibiotics for a longer period of time. If you're getting acute bacterial prostatitis frequently, you need to be cautious with long-term antibiotic use, as bacteria can become resistant to them. It can mess with your healthy gut bacteria AKA microbiome (more on which later).

Frequent infections can also create adhesions and scars around pelvic organs and surrounding tissues, not to mention that your pelvic floor muscles tense up as a protective mechanism. This needs to be addressed physically to avoid the aftermath of overactive pelvic floor muscles (again, more later on this topic).

IS IT AN INFECTION?

I'd recommend getting in touch with a urologist or functional medicine doctor specializing in urologic health. It's always wise to make sure there isn't anything more serious going on. If you're in the clear on the big stuff, ask for a two- or four-glass Meares-Stamey test before taking the antibiotics route. These tests involve getting samples of your prostate fluid and urine to rule out a 'true' bacterial infection.

The most costly yet clinically effective is the two-glass Meares-Stamey test where they take samples of mid-stream urine and post-prostate-massage urine. Studies show this test is 96% effective in correctly identifying a bacterial infection. They look at the samples under a microscope checking for white blood cells (WBCs) and any abnormal bacteria. If WBCs are present, it could mean an bacterial infection. *But* it's also completely normal to have a few WBCs in prostatic fluid. If there are a lot seen under the microscope, the sample is sent for further analysis. If the results come back positive, it's a green light to treat with antibiotics.

Many of the guys I've seen in clinic have never had their prostate fluids checked to rule out infection, but were treated with antibiotics anyway. Here's why that's a problem. What happens is you'll feel good for a short period of time because all antibiotics have a pain-relieving effect, but then the symptoms would return, sometimes even worse than before. It's important that the provider you're seeing doesn't just mask your symptoms by throwing a bunch of meds at you. This kind of treatment is like throwing spaghetti at a brick wall. Nothing really sticks.

Bottom line, antibiotics don't cure non-bacterial persistent pelvic pain.

AND WHAT IF IT'S NOT AN INFECTION?

If you don't have an active infection, like in 95% of cases, it's Type III chronic non-bacterial prostatitis (with or without inflammation), otherwise known as chronic pelvic pain syndrome (CPPS).

Eek! I promised never to use the word chronic, didn't I? Why the difference in these two names though? The NIH changed the name of this category from prostatitis to pelvic pain or CPPS, because the symptoms that you experience might not be coming from your prostate at all. And in my experience, this is often true. Oftentimes, the symptoms you're experiencing are coming from a combination of stress, overactive pelvic floor muscles, anxiety over the issue and not knowing what to do about it, your beliefs and thoughts about pain, social taboos, or even religious views about your private parts. Don't let that word 'inflammation' fool you into thinking this isn't stress- or anything else related. Most often, the presence of inflammation doesn't have a direct correlation to the severity or number of symptoms you experience.

WHAT DOES IT FEEL LIKE?

Given CPPS covers so many potential categories, what does it even feel like? Persistent pelvic pain can include:

- Groin pain
- Tailbone or butt pain
- Burning or sharp pain at the tip, shaft, or base of the penis
- Pain during or after ejaculation
- Pain during or after urination
- Ache in rectum
- Feeling of pressure in the prostate or rectum
- Pain while sitting
- Having to pee every hour
- Abdominal pain
- Testicle pain
- Pain between scrotum and anus
- Lower back pain
- Pain during sex

- ❯ Finding it impossible to sleep through the night without waking up to pee
- ❯ Feeling like you don't empty your bladder all the way
- ❯ Weak or shy urine stream
- ❯ Discomfort with bowel movements
- ❯ Straining with bowel movements

If you're experiencing any of the symptoms listed above, keep reading.

When your family jewels aren't feeling good, what starts to happen? Anxiety, fear, depression and despair settle in, especially if you've had these symptoms for years without a cure. It's enough to scare anyone sh*tless.

Studies report that men with persistent pelvic pain have greater rates of depression and a poorer quality of life overall. And I'm not surprised. When your genitals aren't working like you think they should, the definition of your manhood is at stake. I mean, how often do you talk about your junk to guys in the locker room? Probably never, right? Guys just don't talk about these things, which makes them feel more isolated, vulnerable, and alone when dealing with pelvic pain.

The result? Relationships with family, friends, and partners suffer and social isolation kicks in. The same study that found those men with pelvic pain had higher rates of depression also found their partners had greater rates of pain during sex too. Interesting.

NO MORE FUN IN THE BOOM-BOOM ROOM

When you're in pain, the last thing you want to think about is sex. So it's no wonder sexual trouble is part of the persistent pelvic pain package that you didn't sign up for. Your penis doesn't have a mind of its own and won't just get an erection upon command. Sorry to burst your bubble!

Let's say, for example, you're a 26-year-old dude with burning pain at the tip of your penis, and every time you ejaculate, you get this terrible gnawing ache in your crotch. You don't have any pain getting an erection or during intercourse but you have more and more trouble 'getting it up' and now you're freaking out. You get increasingly frustrated and are worried that you're not 'normal.'

What really went on when you were trying to get it on? Were you scared about performing? Anxious that you'll be in agony for the next couple of days after sex? How's your self-esteem? Worried that your partner's going to find out something's 'wrong' with you? These are real thoughts by real guys just like you.

The NIH surveyed 488 men and found that 74% had ejaculatory pain at some point during their three-month study. It's common to experience sexual problems while having pelvic pain. Unfortunately, sexual issues wreak havoc on your confidence, relationship with yourself and your partner, even causing anxiety that impacts other aspects of your life. We'll talk more about thoughts, pain and the mind in a later chapter, but for now here are a few common sexual problems that you could be experiencing along with your persistent pelvic pain:

- Low libido
- Trouble keeping an erection
- Difficulty with orgasm
- Low volume ejaculate
- Premature ejaculation
- Pain with or after ejaculation
- Performance anxiety
- Hard-flaccid – the penis feels hard or rigid when it's in a flaccid state

WHERE THE HELL DID THIS PAIN COME FROM?

It's been said that up to 50% of men have symptoms of pelvic pain at some point in their lives accounting for over 2 million outpatient visits per year in the United States. There are lots of theories going around about persistent pelvic pain, none of which has been entirely proven. Most are just speculation based on anecdotal evidence or common features seen in research or clinic.

POTENTIAL CAUSES OF PELVIC PAIN:

- ❯ Abdominal or pelvic surgery
- ❯ Stress
- ❯ History of sexual abuse
- ❯ Trauma to the pelvis or genitals (falls, high impact sports, crazy sexcapades)
- ❯ Infection
- ❯ Compulsive orgasm (keyword compulsive!) to fight depression or anxiety
- ❯ Prolonged sitting or cycling
- ❯ Tight or overactive pelvic floor muscles
- ❯ Constipation
- ❯ Hemorrhoids
- ❯ Poor posture and muscle imbalance
- ❯ Spinal cord and nerve root compression
- ❯ Lack of blood flow to the pelvis
- ❯ Digestive disorders like IBS, Crohn's disease

No matter what crazy stuff you've read on the internet, you didn't get pelvic pain from watching porn or masturbating. It's worth knowing as well, in most cases, men with pelvic pain don't have an STD. I'd be super cautious with what you read on the internet because it can serve to make you paranoid. I suggest putting your worries aside; they're only making matters worse.

Okay, enough of the background jibberish. It's time for the fun stuff! Getting to know your privates.

CHAPTER 2

THE LOWDOWN DOWN BELOW

Urethra.

Coccyx.

Fascia.

What?!

Bet you're glad you signed up for this lesson!

The pelvis is made up of bony and muscular parts, including all the stuff on the inside like ligaments, organs, fascia, nerves and blood vessels. You know those muscles down there that keep you from pooping in your pants during those deep kettlebell squats you do at the gym? Yeah, so those make up your pelvic floor. If you think of the pelvis like a large cereal bowl, the pelvic floor muscles make up the bottom of the bowl extending from your pubic bone to your tailbone.

PELVIC FLOOR 101

Now we've located these crucial muscles, I'm going to take you through a quick anatomy lesson focusing on the importance of your pelvic floor, because there's more to your genitals than a cock and balls.

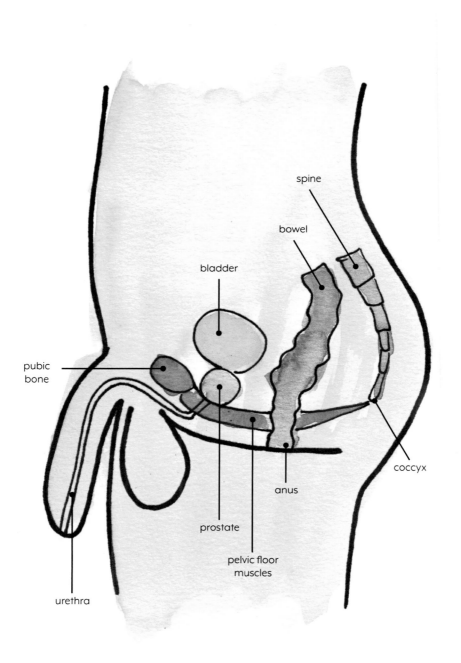

spine

bowel

bladder

pubic
bone

prostate

pelvic floor
muscles

anus

coccyx

urethra

The pelvic floor muscles play a highly important role in your everyday functions, like pooping, peeing, and sex. I call these functions the 5 'S'es.

SPHINCTERIC CONTROL: The pelvic floor muscles clamp down on the tubes that empty your bladder and bowel to keep you continent. They relax when you pee or poop.

SUPPORT: They are the 'foundation' of your body. Their job is to support your abdominal and pelvic organs. They work with your breathing muscle to balance your body's pressure system. For example, when you cough or sneeze, the pelvic floor muscles reflexively tighten to oppose the extra pressure coming down from your belly into your pelvis.

STABILITY: Pelvic floor muscles work together to stabilize your back, pelvis, hips, and legs. They are constantly adjusting to your activity and are working around the clock.

SEXUAL APPRECIATION: Yes, you read that right. Your pelvic floor muscles help with orgasm, getting an erection, keeping an erection, and ejaculation.

SUMP PUMP: Just like with any plumbing, you've got to have good flow down there. When you orgasm and ejaculate, it helps pump out fluid and remove waste improving pelvic blood flow and prostatic pressures. Orgasms also help release feel-good hormones, which can help you get better sleep. If you don't drain the main vein so to say, fluid can build up, so it's healthy to flush out the old stuff once in a while.

There are three layers of muscle groups that make up the pelvic floor. We're going to start from the outermost layer and dive deeper to the innermost layer. Don't worry about pronouncing the names correctly. All you need to know is that these tiny muscles exist and why they're important.

OUTERMOST LAYER:

- Bulbospongiosus
- Ischiocavernosus
- Superficial transverse perineal
- External anal sphincter

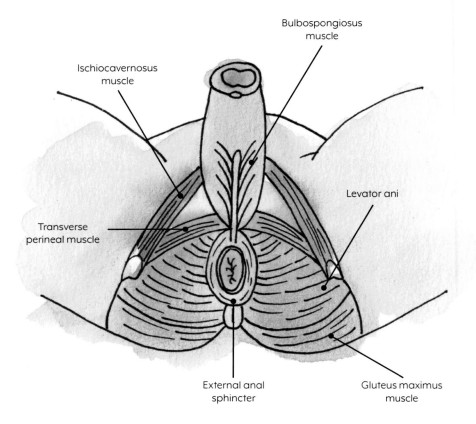

This group of muscles helps with orgasm, ejaculation, urination function (emptying of the urethra) and bowel function. Imagine those times when you need to fart but you're in an elevator full of people; the external anal sphincter helps keep that fart in until you're safe to let loose.

Contrary to what you might think, the penis is actually soft tissue. And it's porous, sorta like a sponge. It's made this way so blood can fill the penis during erection and easily drain after ejaculation. It has

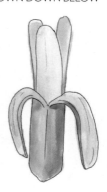

attachments to the bony part of your pelvis and shares connections with the outer and middle layers of the pelvic floor muscles. Next time you peel a banana stick your finger right through the top.

It should split into three pieces. Two pieces on the outside, one on the inside. That's how your penis is structured! Like a hot dog in the middle of the bun. Okay, I'm having too much fun. Moving on...

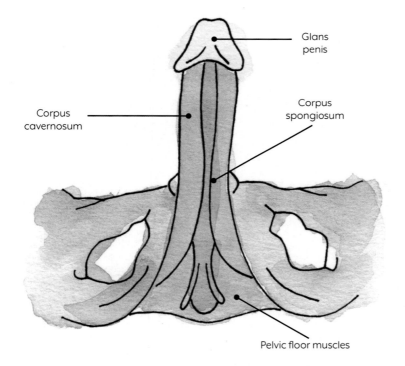

Glans penis

Corpus cavernosum

Corpus spongiosum

Pelvic floor muscles

MIDDLE LAYER:

- ❯ Deep transverse perineal
- ❯ Sphincter urethrae
- ❯ Compressor urethrae
- ❯ Perineal membrane (fibrous connective tissue that separates the middle layer from the outermost layer)

This group adds support to control peeing, has connections with your six-pack abs, and helps stabilize the pelvis and spine during movement. The perineal membrane will be an important landmark for self-treatment described later on.

DEEPEST AND INNERMOST LAYER:

- ❯ Pubococcygeus
- ❯ Puborectalis
- ❯ Iliococcygeus
- ❯ Coccygeus

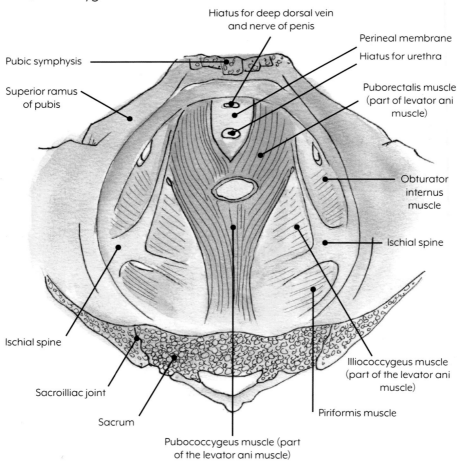

Hiatus for deep dorsal vein and nerve of penis

Perineal membrane

Pubic symphysis

Hiatus for urethra

Superior ramus of pubis

Puborectalis muscle (part of levator ani muscle)

Obturator internus muscle

Ischial spine

Ischial spine

Illiococcygeus muscle (part of the levator ani muscle)

Sacroilliac joint

Piriformis muscle

Sacrum

Pubococcygeus muscle (part of the levator ani muscle)

The diagram shows the innermost layer of the pelvic floor, as viewed from the top. Imagine if I sliced you in half at your waist line and took the top off. What you'd see is the bottom of that cereal bowl I mentioned earlier.

Together, this group of muscles is called the levator ani group, which literally means to 'lift the anus.' These muscles support the pelvic organs (bladder, prostate, and rectum) and help you poop. These tiny little muscles are marathon runners. Their endurance is necessary to help you breathe, poop, walk, and hold up your organs. They've got to keep it all together!

KEGELS AREN'T JUST FOR CHICKS!

Checking in with your body is a good self-assessment practice. So now you know where your pelvic floor muscles are and what they do, can you find them? Let me give you a hint. You'll be able to tell from the outside, ahem, how they're hangin'. Let me walk you through it.

Start by standing naked in front of a mirror. Don't be shy. This is the best feedback you can get.

Next, lift your 'nuts to your guts', meaning try to lift the base of your penis… without using your hands. Or you can think about it as shortening the base of your penis and tightening around the anus like you're stopping the flow of urine or holding back a fart. Or another way of putting it is to 'flick' your penis up and down. And no, I don't mean doing the helicopter!

Did you manage it? How did it feel? What did you see?

When you contract your pelvic floor muscles, the penis moves up and in, the anus lifts and closes, and the testicles slightly lift. When you let go, all parts should move back down to their original position in one smooth transition. There should be a nice visible range of motion with no other muscles helping out. If you're doing it correctly, no-one should be able to tell you're doing them, except for you.

COMMON MISTAKES WITH KEGELS:

❯ Squeezing your butt cheeks

❯ Squeezing your thighs

❯ Tightening your abs

❯ Holding your breath

❯ Pushing down

❯ Giving 100% all the time. Too much of a good thing can lead to overactive or 'tight' pelvic floor muscles which could make symptoms like constipation and pain worse.

Notice what your pelvic floor muscles are doing.

❯ If you're doing a pelvic floor contraction and your dangly bits aren't moving very far, you might have tight pelvic floor muscles which don't let you contract any more or you may need to improve your overall awareness of these muscles.

❯ Perhaps you find yourself contracting your muscles correctly, but have a difficult time relaxing. If so, this might be a sign of tight pelvic floor muscles too.

❯ Alternatively, you might find yourself doing the complete opposite, which means you're bearing or pushing down instead of lifting your pelvic floor muscles.

Being able to perform a pelvic floor contraction correctly can be difficult if you lack awareness about your pelvic floor muscles, but being able to identify your pelvic floor is critical for everything else that's coming up. So stick with it! I'm walking you through these steps in so much detail because being in tune with what you're feeling down there is an important way to self-assess and start making positive progress.

Do you remember the song *Dem Bones*? You know the one that goes…

The back bone connected to the thigh bone,
The thigh bone connected to the knee bone,
The knee bone connected to the leg bone…

Here's the (not so) subliminal message: it's all connected!

The same goes for the pelvic floor muscles. In fact, your hip, back, leg, abdominal muscles, and diaphragm (breathing muscle) all have intimate connections with the pelvic floor. If you want to be successful at treating your pelvic pain, you've got to look at the big picture and not just focus on the part that hurts.

THE DIAPHRAGM-PELVIC-FLOOR CONNECTION

The diaphragm is a dome-shaped muscle that sits underneath your ribcage. It directly connects with your abdominal muscles, ribs, and lower back. It also has connections with vital organs like your liver, lungs and stomach. Nerves that help regulate the calming part of your nervous system connect to the diaphragm and feed back information to an area of the brain called the amygdala, which is responsible for emotions, memory, and fear. This means your diaphragm and breathing pattern can influence your pain perception, emotions and experiences.

During diaphragmatic breathing, A.K.A. deep belly breathing, when you breathe in, the pelvic floor muscles lengthen; then when you breathe out, the pelvic floor muscles return to their natural resting position. Your pelvic muscles affect your breathing and they need to work properly to help control pressure change and fluid flow in the body. Since muscles of your pelvic floor attach to the prostate directly, tight and overactive pelvic floor muscles could lead to a change in prostate fluid flow and prostate mobility. Congestion due to poor fluid flow might mimic inflammation on diagnostic tests.

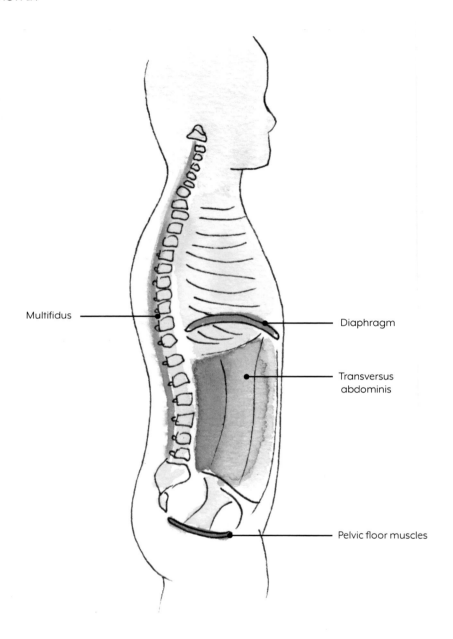

Multifidus

Diaphragm

Transversus abdominis

Pelvic floor muscles

I can't emphasize enough how it's all connected!

Okay, anatomy lesson over. Let's hit the next topic: your brain.

CHAPTER 3

YOUR BODY ON YOUR MIND

You know that feeling you get when you whack your funny bone? I've done it a bunch of times. Does it send me cross-eyed? Sure. Do I know it's going to go away after I shake it off? Yup, no biggie.

Here's the thing about pelvic pain that I really want you to know more than anything else in this book. Pain in the pelvis isn't permanent. Let me repeat that. Despite what doctors tell you, despite what you read on the internet, pain in the pelvis is not permanent.

We all experience pain. Aches and niggles are a normal part of life. Pain doesn't always mean you're in danger or being threatened.

Okay, deep breath. I'm gonna take it a step further. I want you to start thinking of pain as a gift. Now, I know what you're thinking. *Whoa, wait a second. You want me to think about this pain in my ass that I've had for the past eight years as a gift? You're crazy.*

Maybe a little, but not about this. Trust me.

If I'm crazy, how do you explain this? In 2014, the Huffington Post published an article 'Knife Falls From Sky Into Chinese Man's Head.' In it, a Chinese man was casually strolling the block, when out of nowhere, a knife fell into his head. He said he felt 'a very heavy weight' but it wasn't until a bystander pointed out that a knife was stuck in his head that the pain went from feeling just 'heavy' to excruciating.

Luckily, he turned out alright, but the point of telling you this story here is to demonstrate that the sensations you feel are based on the context of the situation and your perception of what's happening to you. For the Chinese man, he was enjoying his walk until someone spoiled it for him telling him he had a knife stuck in his head. His mind had been changed by the information.

Dr. David Butler and Professor Lorimer Moseley, clinical pain scientists, wrote a fantastic book called *Explain Pain*, which I highly recommend reading. You can get a copy at www.noigroup.com/en/Product/EP-BII. Many of my patients' pain levels reduce just by reading this book. And actually, there's research to support that educating a person about their pain, alongside any relevant exercises, relieves the pain better than any medication currently used to treat persistent pain.

THE BRAIN ON PAIN

With persistent pain, the central nervous system (your brain and spinal cord) play an important role in controlling how you feel. According to the International Association for the Study of Pain, pain is described as 'an unpleasant sensory and emotional experience' in response to 'actual or potential tissue damage.' The pain that you feel isn't just experienced in the tissues; it's actually created in the brain *first*.

There's two types of pain that your brain interprets. One is called nociceptive pain, which is a response to a painful stimulus coming from an organ or tissue. For example, if you stepped on a nail or had a knife fall out of the sky and stab you in the skull like our Chinese friend, you would know about it. The second is neuropathic pain, which is pain that is generated by the central nervous system. Neuropathic pain is most commonly associated with persistent pain where your nervous system gets riled up and sensitive to even the slightest information it receives despite whether or not actual tissue injury is present.

But it's not all in your head. Your body parts have sensors (detectors). These sensors send electrical impulses up to your brain for processing. For example, when you're talking it up with your buddies, what's allowing you to hear what they're saying? You might've said your ear and this is partially true. Your ear is a receptacle for sound to tunnel through, creating vibrations that stimulate little hair cells, exciting the nerves of your inner ear. This sends electrical signals to your brain to interpret those vibrations into words that you can actually understand. Fascinating, right?! Well, the same goes for the sensations that you feel in the body.

Those little sensors are found everywhere: in your ligaments, joints, muscles, hair cells, bone, blood vessels, nerves, organs. The list goes on and on. These sensors respond to temperature, touch, pressure, stretch, movement, smell, sight, thoughts, stress, noise. Anything can be a trigger. They're the same sensors that send messages to your brain signaling danger. Just like your brain interprets the sound that comes into your ear, it also interprets 'danger' messages so that it can protect you. Potential dangers can be anything that you perceive as a threat. They can be physical like a snake bite or they can be emotionally driven like the thought of being turned down for a first date.

Not all danger messages are harmful or hurtful. How you interpret these messages is based on a hodgepodge of factors, including:

- Past experiences
- Environment
- Beliefs
- Thoughts
- Values
- Understanding and knowledge
- Safety
- Current situation
- Expectations
- Perspective
- What healthcare providers told you
- Social taboos
- Religious views

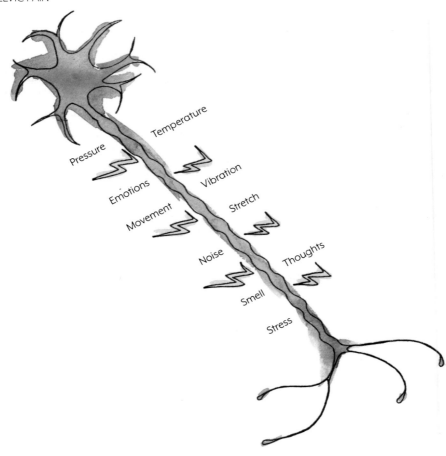

I say '*you* interpret…' because, well, your brain is you!

With persistent pain, the tissues have long since healed but the message in your brain stays the same: that you're 'in danger.' When you have ongoing pain, the signals to your body from your brain get stronger, making the signal sharper. Pain always wants to know what's going on, so it's only natural for danger sensors to sprout and recruit other neighboring tissues to join in on the conversation; this means your pain might feel like it's playing tricks on you. First it's here, then it's there, jumping around all over the place. Pain and muscle tension respond to a 'perceived' threat but that doesn't necessarily mean being directly in harm's way.

My advice here is get a new mantra: I'm sore but I'm safe.

THOUGHTS AND THE VICIOUS CYCLE OF CATASTROPHIZING

Ever heard a voice in your head telling you something like, 'This pain's never going to go away'? *Yes!*

You're not alone. Negative thoughts and worry can run riot through your head when you've got persistent pain. What you might not know is that you're shooting yourself in the foot every time you let these thoughts get out of control. As we've already touched on, pain can worsen just by thinking about a perceived threat. You've watched a horror movie, right? Remember the escape scene from *The Silence of the Lambs*, for example, where Hannibal Lecter bites off the prison guard's face? I'm willing to bet you knew what was coming... Didn't it make your heart beat just a little quicker and your muscles tense up scooting to the edge of your seat? The reason I mention this is to show you how you don't have to be in any actual real direct danger for your brain to interpret it as such, causing your body to respond in a protective way. The threat alone can create a pain sensation without any actual tissue damage or injury.

If horror movies aren't your thing, how about this story? I once asked my husband if he or his friends had ever performed self-inflicted torture to their testicles, just mucking around. He remembered a time where he and his mate messed about with a BB gun, shooting each other with air at close range. His friend Mike thought it would be a fun idea to test out the gun at close range, pointing the gun to his balls. Unfortunately, it wasn't just air that came out that time. One black and blue ball later, Mike was jumping around with tears in his eyes at the horrific pain that followed. Did you just make your *oh-sh*t-that's-gotta-hurt* face when reading that? Maybe even felt the urge to protect your own family jewels? That's your body's response to an anticipated threat. The thought of a BB gun shooting you in your nads makes you flinch and protect them. Get where I'm going with this?

Pain is a protective response that might be making the tissues in your body hypersensitive to touch or movement. Your thoughts and beliefs about your pain can either be liberating or give you more anxiety. Depends on your perspective. The longer and more persistent those negative thoughts loop around in your mind, the more the brain will adapt and create stronger, more powerful output signals to the site of your pain. Eventually, other neighboring areas corresponding to different parts of your body in the brain will also start getting stimulated, even though that part of your body or organ system is completely healthy.

Researchers discovered that the combination of long-standing pelvic pain with this 'catastrophizing' actually changes the brain structure and function over time. The front left part of your brain deals with positive feelings like hope and joy. The front right part of your brain deals with negative emotions like anxiety and sadness. The research found that those who have persistent pain have reduced activity in the left part of the brain and increased activity in the right. That means feeling more down in the dumps, socially withdrawn and hopeless when long-standing pain combines with the negative thought behavior already mentioned.

Stress and anxiety (such as that which can be related to persistent pain) can even shrink your brain. Another study showed that the parts of the brain that deal with receiving sensory information from your pelvis have higher activity, which makes what you're feeling down there more sensitive than it should be. These brain changes impact the processing and integration of sensory information from your pelvic floor. And if your thoughts, behaviors, past experiences, stress, and fears continue to haunt you, it's no wonder why your brain keeps telling you that your private parts are in danger. Naturally, your muscles tense up, get tighter and impact the overall health of your pelvic floor.

What's more amazing is that research has shown that the parts of your brain controlling movement also influence the adrenal glands. The adrenal glands located on top of your kidneys are responsible for secreting stress hormones especially during times of 'fight or flight.' Sympathetic activation impacting the control of stress is also located in the same area of the brain. Even the *thought* of you being angry or sad will activate the sympathetic centers in the brain and influence the adrenal glands.

The replaying of events – ahem, like the frustrations of having to deal with pelvic pain – also affect the same area, further driving your stress response. So do like the tennis players do and 'let the match point go.'

The opposite occurs in another motor area of the brain associated with the 'reward system.' This lights up during mindful meditation, the practice of 'letting go' and core muscle exercise. These areas, when lit, have the opposite effect on your adrenal glands, decreasing the stress response. I just love science, don't you?

Stress has been shown to make concentration and everyday function exhausting. No wonder pelvic pain can be draining and make you so tired all the time. The energy you're putting into thinking about your pain is tiring you out, especially since thoughts are actual physical nerve impulses.

But if your thoughts have the ability to create pain, they also have the ability to get you out of pain. Which is the good news. Enter the autonomic nervous system, your body's regulator.

GETTING ON YOUR NERVES

If you hadn't figured it out already, your nerves are important because they make up the communication highway between the body and the brain. The central nervous system is what I like to call the 'big boss' and this boss works two shifts: 'rest and digest' and 'fight or flight.' These two states collectively make up your autonomic nervous system (ANS), which is responsible for managing your bodily functions, communicating with your brain and organs, responding to emergency and non-emergency situations. Typically, if there's been an injury, tissues heal within 12 to 16 weeks. Any persisting symptoms aren't necessarily a direct cause of tissue injury; there are other mechanisms at play that we need to investigate. Namely, the thoughts in your head, which we know have an impact on feeling pain.

Think you're maybe dealing with more than just a muscle issue here? Study your thoughts, as they should tip you off. Some thoughts that indicate your mind is in play with your pain could include:

'It seems like the pain is every other day.'

'My pain's never the same. It's always moving around.'

'Nothing helps anymore.'

'My pain gets worse when I'm stressed.'

'The pain comes out of nowhere.'

'When I've got to confront my boss, the pain skyrockets.'

'The pills don't even work. I don't know why I'm taking them.'

'I won't become a (fill in the blank) and I'll never reach my goals'.

'No-one will want me.'

Can you relate to any of those statements? Maybe you've even used some of them in the past? Statements like these are big indicators that the pain is probably not in your tissues anymore. It's more in the nervous system.

Of the two 'states' I identified as making up the central nervous system, the *sympathetic nervous system* is your 'fight or flight' response mechanism. The Mike Tyson of the nerve world. It's the switch that quickly turns on when you need protection or when you're getting ready to jump out of a plane skydiving with your friends.

Adrenaline and cortisol are stress hormones that help protect you. When this fight or flight switch is turned on, your body gets flooded with stress hormones so your gut gets sluggish, your heart and respiratory rate increase, you sweat bullets, get goosebumps, your energy and power are amped up, and your pelvis makes sure you don't have the urge to poop or pee while fighting for your life ('cause that would be bad). These are all important reactions when you're actually in danger but what happens when your body goes through this on a daily basis? When you don't come down from that high-stress rollercoaster ride?

Your mind and body suffer from sympathetic overload, releasing 'fight or flight' chemical messengers by way of hormones like adrenaline and cortisol that, over time, can affect your immune system, clarity, cognitive function, mood, muscle tone, blood pressure, hormonal function, sleep patterns, digestive system, libido, brain structure... Just to name a few.

Wait a sec?! Did I just suggest a loss in libido from stress?! Yup, I sure did. Cortisol, the stress hormone, acts as a protector in some ways. Cortisol helps turn off inflammation in the body, for one. However, under longer bouts of stress, the immune cells become resistant to cortisol, sending your immune response into overdrive. Great to have for the short term, but not so nice under prolonged conditions. Inflammation, anyone?

You might be wondering what that mechanism has to do with pain in the pelvis. Well, cortisol levels have been shown to be higher in men with persistent pelvic pain than men without pelvic pain. Meaning elevated levels of cortisol can impact tissue healing, sleep, memory, depression, anxiety, immunity, and your sex drive.

You'll be happy to hear, though, that for all there is a Mike Tyson of the nerve world, there is also a Mahatma Gandhi. The *parasympathetic nervous system* is the 'rest and digest' response system. When this switch is turned on, it lets you digest that burger you just ate, relaxes your heart rate and breathing, stimulates the production of calming chemical messengers like serotonin (the 'happy' chemical of the brain that is produced mostly in your gut), relaxes your muscles, and allows your bladder and bowel to relax so that you can take care of business.

When your body is unable to come back down from an overly aroused nervous system, it begins to work on overdrive which can exacerbate your current pain experience. When your body is at rest, however, it has the ability to heal itself as well as stimulate normal bodily functions in order for you to combat the demands of life, including sex. Woohoo! Now we're getting somewhere.

EFFECTS OF PROLONGED PAIN AND STRESS ON OTHER SYSTEMS

Of course, it's a little more complex than just positive-thinking and resting, because it's not just the nervous system at play. (It's all connected, remember!) There are multiple body systems that all work together so that you can function at your best. They're constantly communicating and we're designed so that, if one system is underperforming for some reason, another one has to take up the slack.

Pain can affect any of these systems:

- Hormone
- Immune
- Nervous
- Respiratory
- Emotional
- Muscular
- Brain

As we've seen in the last section, when you're physically or emotionally stressed, your body activates that 'fight or flight' response in the nervous system to protect you. Multiple systems are involved when it comes to protecting you from a perceived threat or an actual threat. The effect of this on other systems is worth noting.

Let's start with the immune system. Under prolonged stress, your cells receive a signal to promote inflammation. Eventually, chemical changes can affect your immune system too by producing more inflammatory chemical messengers. This can even 'wake up' old aches and pains just by tapping into the brain's tissue memory bank.

And what about the muscular system? You won't be surprised that, as always, it's all connected and related. The muscular system doesn't get let off the hook when we're talking about prolonged stress either. It's no coincidence that we call stressed-out controlling people 'uptight' or 'anal retentive.' When you're under stress, a bit anxious, wired and tired, your pelvic floor reacts in the same way.

Recognizing when and where you hold your tension in your body is key to start letting it go. Studies have proven that your emotions affect your muscle tension and ability to relax, because the body and the mind are so intimately connected. When you're under stress, you unconsciously start developing 'holding patterns' or tension within the body. For you, maybe it so happens to be in the pelvic floor.

Persistent or prolonged holding patterns can lead to altered pelvic floor muscle function, restriction around blood vessels and nerves, and poor movement of pelvic organs. After a while, your body starts to have trouble compensating for this imbalance and will let you know like, 'Hello, I'm talking to you,' AKA pain. If ignored long enough, this message will get louder and louder, until it's screaming bloody murder to get your attention. If this was your hamstring muscle, for example, you probably wouldn't think much about it, but it's your penis we're talking about so naturally tensions start to rise.

On it goes... Louder and louder... Creating more anxiety, more pain, more anxiety, more pain. This perpetuating fear can trap you in a vicious pain-tension cycle. Just another example of how your thoughts can create pain. (Hint: using WebMD to self-diagnose isn't the smartest idea if you want to get out of this anxiety trap.)

The vicious circle goes round and round until you decide it's time to get off. Anxiety is pro-inflammatory and will increase those stress chemical messengers to your brain to stimulate more pain receptors, increasing your sensitivity. It's kinda like a smoke alarm that goes off if you just blow on it. The damn thing goes blaring but there's nothing serious going on. The problem with alarms is they're designed to be sensitive. Just like your fight or flight response.

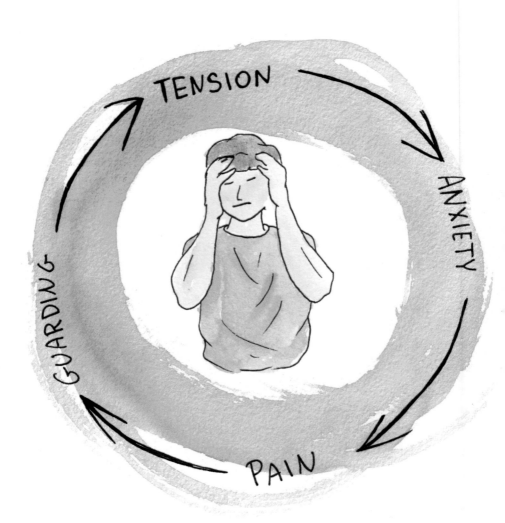

But just as I've mentioned previously and want to reiterate here and now, your pain isn't permanent. If you can turn it on, you can turn it off.

So what's the first step to controlling your tension? Becoming aware of it. It's sometimes hard to bring awareness inside your body when you've been so distracted by the outside. I've had patients walking into my clinic with their shoulders up to their ears from so much tension. When I ask them to relax their shoulders, they'll say, 'But they are relaxed.' Your body creates a new threshold, a new level of 'dealing with it' and eventually you get so used to it that you forget what 'normal' or letting go feels like.

Yet awareness and breaking the tension-anxiety-pain-guarding cycle is possible. All it takes is patience, commitment, and a little TLC.

CHAPTER 4

TRAIN YOUR BRAIN

Athlete Michael Phelps wouldn't have won 28 career Olympic medals without challenging and changing his mindset. Most athletes train with sports psychologists that focus on mental rehearsing, cognitive behavioral therapy, and mindfulness based stress reduction. This form of psychology focuses on mindful awareness without judgement, which changes the way you think and react in certain situations. Changing the way you think about your pelvic pain is essential to getting better.

It's not uncommon for men with pelvic pain to feel hopeless, angry, depressed and frustrated about their symptoms. In fact, anxiety and depression usually go hand in hand with men who experience pelvic pain.

And who could blame you if you're feeling this way? We're talking about your manhood, the one thing that (at least according to everything men are ever told) defines your masculinity. Problems with the plumbing would make anyone worried and anxious. But what happens when these thoughts rattle around in your brain longer than you'd like? Repetitive catastrophizing thoughts like, 'I'll never get better,' 'It's just going to get worse,' or 'I'll live like this for the rest of my life' light up danger messengers in the brain making the signal stronger and more in-your-face.

Going to see a psychologist doesn't mean you're crazy, depressed, or have to sit there talking about feelings. Instead think about it as mental coaching. It's about training your brain to get into the right state of mind, just like the pros do.

OWNING YOUR PELVIC PAIN

Let's start with the first helpful mind trick to tackle your pelvic pain: owning it.

Nobody wants to 'own' their pelvic pain or any pain for that matter, but there's some truth to the benefits behind why you should. Pelvic pain doesn't happen overnight. It might seem like it did. Yet in most cases, it's a build-up of events that causes the body to make a screeching halt and say, 'Hey, pay attention to me!' It's your body telling you that something has to change, whether that's lifestyle, thoughts, behaviors, or your annoying boss. (Yep, seriously!)

The body is constantly trying to adjust and compensate for the daily grind that it goes through. Some people are better than others at finding that 'life balance.' But it's okay if you're not one of them. Just like you can beef up your biceps, you can also strengthen your brain by shifting your focus and attention to change the way you feel.

In conventional medicine, the approach is more 'find it and fix it', which means you take something of a passive role in your health. Men with pelvic pain often end up seeing a bunch of medical providers searching for that one 'magic cure', only to be left more frustrated and hopeless. Most of the patients I see want to know how they can take care of the problem themselves or at least self-manage it, so they feel more in control of their health. Relying on others to 'fix' you will lead you to a dead end.

This is why owning it is the first step to taking back control. It means being proactive, not passive. And it's a huge shift in mindset that's going to help change those unhelpful thoughts.

So... it's okay to own it!

BUT WHY ME?

As annoying as it is to have pelvic pain, you could and should take it one step further and even be thankful for it. *Whaaa?!* You read that right. Let's thank your body for giving you the heads-up that something's wrong. It's the subtle hints we forget to pay attention to that lead up to a major catastrophe like pelvic pain. Your body gives out warning signs to nudge you to take better care of yourself. In such a busy world, those signals often get lost in the crowd.

Taking better care of yourself isn't just about a healthy diet and exercising, because let's face it, even some of the craziest health nuts I know get sick, including me. We all have our 'weak spots.' For me, it's sinus congestion and allergies. Stress impacts all your body's systems, but some are stronger than others and the wimpy systems end up getting the short end of the stick.

Dr. Lissa Rankin MD, a body-mind doctor from California, asks her patients two questions during their appointment: 'What do you think might lie at the root of your illness?' and 'What does your body need in order to heal?'

You might say something like, 'I need to lose weight,' 'I need to exercise more,' or 'I have to stop eating donuts for breakfast,' but most of the time it's the elephant in the room that you avoid at all costs, like, 'I hate my job,' 'I'm not in love with my partner anymore,' 'I need a break,' 'I hate where I live,' 'I don't know what to do with my life,' 'I need more fun,' 'I don't have friends,' 'My mom left when I was nine years old,' and so on and so on.

Your thoughts and emotions get stored in your tissues so that your mind doesn't fry. I love the way Dr. Rankin puts it. 'The body doesn't fuel how we live our lives. Instead, it is a mirror of how we live our lives.'

So I challenge you right now to ask yourself those two questions:

What do I think is the root cause of my pelvic pain?
and
What does my body need in order for it to heal?

It's okay if you don't have the answer right away. Remember, healing from pelvic pain is a journey and finding the answer to these questions might be part of the quest.

SHHH, BE QUIET!

Quieting down overactive and tight pelvic floor muscles takes time, patience, and commitment. Imagine walking around with your biceps flexed as if you were showing off your guns for two years straight. How do you think that arm will start feeling? After one day? A month? A year? Okay, I'm exaggerating the point, but it's to explain what happens to the pelvic floor muscles when they're too tight, overactive and tense over a long period of time. The muscles stop working well, and the blood flow, nerves and organs start to adapt to the current situation. Tight or shortened pelvic floor muscles don't allow for normal pelvic floor function and this results in disrupting the ebb and flow, not only of the pelvis but also of other parts of your body. Because remember, it's all connected!

You probably weren't even aware that those muscles existed until they started talking back to you. And that's the thing. It's likely that there was a lack of body awareness and intuition over a long period, so the subtle messages of your body were ignored. So first things first. Let's get quiet enough to know what that part of your body feels like on a subtle level, rather than just fixating on the pain. Learn to recognize when those muscles are tight or relaxed. Then you can control them more efficiently.

Learning to relax these muscles helps:

- Improve oxygen to the tissues
- Improve nutrition and blood flow
- Heal tissues
- Get rid of waste products
- Improve immune system filtration flow (lymphatic system)

❯ With pooping and peeing more easily
❯ With gut motility

Now, don't get me wrong. Letting go might feel a bit weird.

I had a patient once tell me that he felt 'weird' letting go of his butt. After being a butt-gripper for 10 years, who could blame him? It's been one of his holding patterns for years and his body just got used to being that way. It's a lot of work training your mind to shift the focus from outside of your body back into your body, especially when pain's involved. That means it's perfectly normal to feel uncomfortable in your own skin during this process of letting go.

We all go through 'growing pains' when our cells start to change. It's called *resistance*. Whenever you're trying to change a behavior, habit, or whatever else, there's a process that your mind and body go through. It's like that New Year's resolution you set for yourself. 'I'm going to exercise every day for an hour.' Okay great! So January 1st rolls around and you're pumped, ready to take action and rock 'n' roll. The first week you're amped and proud that you've stuck with it for a whole seven days. As soon as that second week hits, it feels like such a drag. Then come the excuses and you're back to where you were last year. Sound familiar? Does for me. Your brain and cells actually go through physical and chemical changes when you're learning a new behavior or changing an old one. Change is hard for anyone and learning to down-train overly tense muscles and an amped up nervous system takes grit.

And some patience…

BUT I WANT IT NOW

So how much time will this take? Well, that depends on your investment. Everyone's situation is different and the time it takes to heal will vary. Pelvic pain didn't happen overnight and it won't go away overnight either. I know this is a hard concept to grasp in a world where instant gratification prevails and you've got answers just seconds away in the palm of your hands. Yet change really does require daily practice and attention to your body's needs. Your perspective contributes to the healing process. You can be in the driver's seat or you can be the passenger. In other words, you can choose to have pain dictate your life or you can take the bull by its horns.

Remember, your thoughts and emotions trigger physical reactions. The harder you try to get rid of the pain, the more resistance your body's going to give you. Trying equals effort and effort equals work. Those pelvic floor muscles have already been overworked and underpaid; no need to keep adding to that cycle. Acceptance and understanding of what you're going through will keep the tension, stress, and anxiety at bay, allowing your body to take the lead and heal.

Your body is a miracle and has the intrinsic ability to heal itself. You just have to trust it. A life without pain is possible.

TEMPER TANTRUMS AWAIT

What's more, there will be ups and downs along the way, even with acceptance. Most people think getting better is a straight and easy road, going from point A to point B. But that's not realistic. Healing is a journey along a winding road. With detours, speed bumps, stops, and panoramic views. Through this process you're given a chance to grow, get out of your comfort zone, push your limits, and see your health and life through a different lens. It's an opportunity to learn more about yourself and take care of yourself so you can reach your highest potential in whatever life has to offer you.

You need to leave space for good days and bad days. Flare-ups are common and nothing to worry about. You're not getting worse and you're not back at square one. Think of it as that resistance analogy I just shared with you. Your body's freaking out because you're trying to change its old ways. Naturally, there will be days where your body's going to throw a temper tantrum and that's perfectly okay. Let it scream and shout, but don't cave into it. It's kinda like that kid at the store you see screaming on the floor for mom to buy him a toy. As uncomfortable and embarrassing as it is for mom, she's not going to cave because the minute she does, little Bobby knows that all he has to do is put on this performance every time he wants something. Same goes for your body.

Oh and remember all that talk about the brain? Don't forget that anything could be a trigger to set off that alarm. Take some time to think about what those triggers might be. Pay attention to how your body is feeling throughout the day and jot it down. You'll most likely find a pattern or theme.

ALL ABOUT CONTEXT

Let's say you're having a week from hell. You're behind on all your projects, the car's giving you trouble, you're eating like sh*t and sleep is nonexistent, you're fighting with your partner, oh and to top it all off, you just found out that you can't have those vacation days. Just an all-round craptastic week. Then you decide, 'Oh screw it, I'm going to masturbate. Gotta have *some* fun this week at least.' But damn, there's a flare-up. Talk about a cock block. This time around it's unbearable, lasting longer than normal. For someone whose nervous system is already on high alert, it's no wonder your alarm bells are going off louder than normal. You've had a hellish week after all.

See, it's all about the context of the situation. Your week was sh*tty, so your body reacts by creating more tension. You get more anxious and less cautious about taking care of yourself. This is completely normal. We all fall off the health bandwagon once in a while.

Now, let's say the opposite were true. Let's say you're having the best week of your life! You got that promotion, you went camping with your friends, you played hockey for the first time in years. And guess what. You felt fine. No flare-ups. This time when you ejaculate, your pain's not nearly as high, almost nonexistent. Surprised? You shouldn't be. It's because of the situation. The week was great, you had some fun. As a result, your mind and body reacted in the same way. Relaxed.

So next time your pain feels worse, take a step back to analyze your life in the recent weeks. What's been going on? Can you identify some possible triggers? The better you get at realizing what makes you and your body tick, the better you'll be able to control them. Awareness is key. The Protectometer app is a great tool you can use to help you discover those triggers. Download it from www.noigroup.com/en/Product/EPHP.

GET THOSE ZZZZS

It doesn't matter if you're a night owl or an early bird, as long as you're getting restful sleep. Your body needs this time to repair and rejuvenate to prepare you for the challenges of the next day. Sleep problems and persistent pain go together like peanut butter and jelly.

Your sleep quality can predict the level of pain you have the following day. For some, the night time is when their pain levels worsen. Why? Theory has it that cortisol, the stress hormone, runs on a circadian rhythm. Normally, it spikes first thing in the morning, dies down, increases midday and then comes back down at night. That means the protective mechanism used in your fight or flight mode – cortisol – is supposed to be lower at night. However, if it's on overdrive through stress, over time cortisol becomes insensitive to inflammation. There comes a point when cortisol doesn't help to reduce inflammation and it will make your symptoms seem like they're much worse, especially during times of fluctuation. For example, during the day, you're distracted, flying high on adrenaline. Come bedtime, though, your ammunition runs low so it's easier for your brain to pay attention to your body including the aches and pains.

Sleep is important because without it your body doesn't rest and repair, continuously perpetuating the stress cycle and making your nervous system more sensitive to the pain response.

GETTING THE BEST OUT OF YOUR SLEEP

It's not only the kiddos that need a bedtime routine. Adults need them too. If you're having a hard time shutting off your brain at night, try to build a better bedtime ritual. Create a more suitable environment to make sure you're getting those zzzs. Too much artificial light can throw off your sleep-wake patterns. Ahem, this includes your computer, phone, and video game screens. So if you're up all night playing video games, you might want to start thinking of some new bedtime habits.

Start by tapping into your current bedtime routine. What does bedtime look like for you? How does your body feel? What are you doing? Do you look forward to sleeping or do you dread it?

According to Dr. Rubin Naiman, a clinical psychologist specializing in integrative sleep and dream medicine, 'Sleep is an experience.' If you're tossing and turning, getting frustrated that you can't fall asleep, this may be a part of the problem. Like accepting your pelvic pain, you need to start accepting your sleeplessness. The anxiety and effort in paying attention to all the things in your life that are 'not going so well' only creates more tension, adrenaline, and anxiety around the very thing you're fighting so hard against. Dr. Naiman suggests, 'Sleep will naturally and gradually begin to seep through when we let go of effort. Relinquishing sleep effort is about letting go of our waking self – our sense of who we believe we are. It's about willingly losing the battle for control of sleep by realizing that falling asleep cannot be controlled. Sleep is, in essence, a free ride for all those who are simply willing to be passengers.'

I'm going to rattle off some tips for better sleep, but remember, you're unique and should customize a routine for your lifestyle. There's no one size fits all.

- Switch off that blue light! Shut down your TV, phone, tablet, or whatever you use for one to two hours before bed.
- If letting go of technology is too hard, try using a blue light filter like F.lux. (justgetflux.com).
- No caffeine or sugary snacks before bedtime.
- Be mindful. Maybe you like journaling? If journaling isn't for you, try meditation. I'm not all against the use of technology. Try listening to a podcast called *Sleep with Me* (sleepwithmepodcast.com) or use meditation apps like Headspace (headspace.com) or Calm (calm.com) to get you sleeping like a baby.
- Take a bath.
- Use your bed for sleep and sexual activity only (no snacking, reading or watching TV).
- Keep your bedroom dark and cool.
- Go to sleep and wake up at the same time every day. This trains your biological clock.
- Don't pump iron right before bed. High impact, adrenaline-pumping exercise energizes your body. Not a good idea if you're having trouble falling asleep.
- If you're going to watch TV, try watching something that's relaxing, fun, and lighthearted. Watching a nail-biter right before bed will flick on your fight and flight response mechanism, which isn't helpful when trying to get some sleep.
- Don't work so hard in the evening. Just like your body, your mind needs a break too.
- Breathe yourself to sleep. Deep belly breathing helps lower your heart rate, decreases tension in muscles, lowers your blood pressure, and stimulates the 'rest and digest' nervous system.
- Go play outside! The more natural sunlight you get, the better your sleep cycle.

MAYBE YOU'RE HORMONAL?

Stay with me here.

In my practice, I've seen a few young guys with pelvic pain show up with low levels of testosterone. This got me thinking: Is there a connection between low T and pelvic pain in men? So I hit the books, researching near and far for the answer. And you know what I came up with? Nothing. Okay, I didn't come up entirely empty-handed but the research about this topic is slim to none.

But I didn't call it quits. I kept digging and put together some of my own thoughts based on the research.

When you suddenly get pain 'down there', a ripple of events most likely happens. You go see an MD, who most likely gives you some antibiotics and then sends you on your merry way. A month or so goes by and you feel a little better with the meds but the pain comes back. So you go back to the doctor and they give you another round of antibiotics... And then another... And another. By now, it's probably been a good seven or eight months, maybe even a year dealing with this nightmare. You're frustrated, pissed, and feeling hopeless. You've seen too many doctors and gotten no answers. You might've been told you're just going to have to live with this for the rest of your life – the ultimate death sentence that sends you over the edge. (No joke doctors are still saying things like this to their patients. It's not their fault. They only know so much and get intimidated by conditions like persistent pelvic pain because they just don't know how to help you. Don't get me wrong. They all have good intentions but they might've just exhausted all the tools in their toolbox.)

Hearing this doesn't mean you should crawl into a dark hole and sulk in your sorrows. It means that there are other wellness professionals with other perspectives that might help you get the results you want. There's hope. Unfortunately, because you're only human, you start doubting your ability to get over this and those negative thoughts looping around and around in your head start controlling your life. The worry. The anxiety. These two life-sucking demons have negative impacts on your overall health and wellbeing. It's no wonder that over half of men with persistent pelvic pain have depression.

Now, remembering that stress and anxiety impact your pain, sleep, hormone, immune and nervous systems, here's what happens next. Thoughts of frequent worry shrink the brain, impacting your ability to think and make decisions. Stress sets off the fight or flight response mechanism of the body. Doing this releases protective chemical hormones like cortisol, adrenaline, norepinephrine to make sure there's balance in the body. So far, so normal. We've gotten to grips with this in previous chapters.

Over time, though, the release of these protective chemicals impacts the pathways that produce your hormones. Cortisol is a thief and will steal or alter the production of other hormones like testosterone, DHEA (which you need for making T), and many other crucial hormonal pathways.

Can low testosterone be the major contributing factor for your symptoms? Most likely not. Very few studies have shown any relationship. One study did suggest that low T symptoms and 'prostatitis-like' symptoms had a connection, but the research was not strong enough to support any claim, admitting 'we believe that T can affect CP/CPPS but only to a limited extent because the cause of CP/CPPS is multifactorial.'

Bottom line: There are too many other systems in play that feed off of each other to create the symptoms you feel.

While there is no evidence linking testosterone to pelvic pain, here's a bit more about testosterone so that you get to know more about your body and use your own judgement. Testosterone levels depend on your age, health, weight, stress, etc. It's normal for testosterone levels to decrease with age. Typically, T levels start declining 1% each year after your hit your mid-30s.

When evaluating what's 'normal', it all depends on you and how you're feeling. Lab values can range anywhere from 250 ng/dL to 1,000 ng/dL. Again, this depends on how you're feeling. For some guys, they feel great at 500 ng/dL. Others feel better with functional T levels at 800 ng/dL. Every dude is different.

COMMON SIGNS AND SYMPTOMS OF LOW T:

- ❯ Unexplained increase in weight
- ❯ Less frequent morning or spontaneous erections
- ❯ Mood swings, irritability
- ❯ Constant fatigue
- ❯ Brain fog
- ❯ Loss in muscle mass
- ❯ Decreased libido

If you're experiencing these symptoms, it might benefit you to check out your reproductive hormone levels *and* your stress hormones. Remember, with persistent pelvic pain it's not uncommon to have altered levels of testosterone, but generally speaking they shouldn't be tanked.

One more thing about T… Testosterone levels aren't just altered by stress. They can fluctuate based on your sleep patterns, diet, inflammation in the body, pain, gut microbiome, use of over-the-counter muscle-building products, or steroids.

I'm putting your mind at rest; there's no evidence to prove that low testosterone is the cause of pelvic pain. As I mentioned before, it's most likely a smorgasbord of events that were brewing over time until your body just couldn't find another loophole other than SOS so that you could start paying attention to your body and current lifestyle.

Which brings me to my next topic. Drumroll please…

CHAPTER 5

A SIGNAL FOR SELF-CARE

Ever feel butterflies in your stomach going out on a first date? Your brain and gut talk to each other. They go back and forth like a two-way highway. Brain-gut, gut-brain. In fact, the gut actually has its own special nervous system separate from the brain and spinal cord. The gut-brain axis regulates the neuro-endocrine (nervous and hormone system) and immune functions. So technically, we're talking about the brain, spinal cord, nervous system and gut all sharing the same plan.

What happens when they all share the same plan? If one goes over the minutes, the entire bill goes up, that's what. This is what happens to the body. If you're under stress, this will signal a cascade of events trickling from the brain to your gut and through the rest of your body, including the gut bacteria. And vice-versa. What you eat and put into your body can alter your gut bacteria and create the same rippling effect up the chain.

WHAT'S ALL THIS ABOUT MY GUT?

Gut bacteria can impact your mood, including anxiety, via neural and hormonal pathways. In fact, a 2016 study showed that gut microbiota could play an important role in identifying CPPS. It showed that *prevotella* – a bacteria mostly found in your gut and oral cavity – was the lowest in men with CPPS. Interestingly enough, *prevotella* may play a role at reducing inflammation and is higher in people who eat a high fiber, high vegetable diet. Go figure! A healthy gut can decrease the inflammation in your body, enhance your mood, strengthen your immune system, and improve your sleep and pain patterns.

Food is powerful medicine without side effects. What you put in your body mirrors how you feel. Processed sugar, fast food, fried foods, caffeine – to name a few – have been proven to worsen inflammation in the body. And inflammation as you now know increases the sensitivity of your pain sensation and weakens your immune system. There's plenty of research to back up your mom's nagging about vitamins when you were a kid. We need things like omega 3 fatty acids, oleic acid (found olive oil, sunflower oil, nuts and meats), vitamins E, B (1,2,6,13), D, magnesium, minerals (copper, selenium, zinc and calcium), antioxidants, carnitine (amino acid). Did you just get a brain freeze? Let me make this simple. Eat. Real. Food.

All of those nutrients that I just listed are found in fruits, veggies, dark leafy greens, beef, chicken, fish, nuts, beans, olive oil... You get the gist. When it comes to healing your body, you've got to consider healing it from the inside out. And the first step is changing the way you eat.

I hope I didn't just make you panic. I know how hard it is to make lifestyle changes, especially when it comes to food. I'm a foodie myself. So let's take the pressure off a bit. If you're not ready to go cold turkey and stop eating pizza four nights a week, start adding some of these foods *into* your diet and slowly eliminate the junk. It's not going to be easy at first. Sugar's more addicting than cocaine. (Research shows 94% of cocaine-dependent rats made the switch to sugar given the choice, even when they had to work harder for it.)

But just because that stuff isn't easy doesn't mean it isn't worth making the switch, because your body is giving you a big fat signal to prioritize self-care.

BLADDER IRRITANTS

So can you drink Red Bull? Umm, no. Even if it's zero sugar and zero calorie. (It doesn't taste good for nothing. It has other crazy stuff in it to make that happen!)

I once had a patient with pelvic pain and urinary urgency come in saying that his urge to pee all the time came back. I asked if he'd done anything to change his diet, stress, or sleep, and he responded that he hadn't. We were 30 minutes into the session and he tells me about how he drank Red Bull trying to pull an all-nighter driving home from a baseball game. Something that wasn't usual for him.

Why am I not surprised the symptoms got worse? Red Bull, soda, coffee, iced tea, and any other sugary sweet beverages can make your bladder go bonkers. Every person is different but typically drinks that make you pee often can exacerbate your symptoms.

Here are other bladder irritants:

- Spicy foods
- Coffee
- Alcohol

And if you still don't believe me that sugar is kryptonite, a 2011 study in the *American Journal of Clinical Nutrition* showed that low to moderate sugar-sweetened beverage consumption promoted inflammation in healthy young men within just three weeks. Even at the lowest dose of 40g/day, changes were seen. And they were being generous with that low dose. According to the American Heart Association, you should consume no more than about 25-37g sugar/day. To put it in perspective, one 12oz can of Coke has 39g of sugar in it! There goes your day's worth.

So heads up! When deciding where to start, make sugar-sweetened soda the first thing to go.

Since we're on the topic of peeing, let's talk about poop. Everybody's favorite!

THE SCOOP ON POOP

If you're hulking it to pop out that turd, we need to talk. Pelvic floor muscles get annoyed when they're repetitively stressed. Since it's their job to stabilize and protect your pelvic organs, it's only natural that they're going to tense up and guard every time you're dropping a deuce.

So how do we fix this problem? Two things: Sit like 'the Thinker' and breathe.

TOILETING POSTURE

How you sit on the toilet affects your pelvic floor muscles. Your rectum *damn near killed 'em*. Get it? Rec-tum as in 'wrecked him.' Okay, just trying to lighten the mood over here, but seriously check yourself before you wreck yourself!

The rectum sits naturally in the pelvis with a 90-degree bend in it, getting help from your pelvic floor muscles to make sure you don't go around pooping yourself. When you sit down on the toilet in an upright posture, these muscles only semi-relax which makes it harder to poop without straining.

The solution? A step stool. Ta-dah!

Before the luxury of toilets, people squatted to poop. Think of the last time you went camping, no Porta-Potty in sight, what did you do? Ass to grass, right?

STEP 1: SQUAT TO DROP
Using a step stool under your feet will help bring the floor closer to you to mimic that optimal position, allowing full relaxation of your pelvic floor muscles and straighter rectum to make the flow flawless.

Rest your forearms on your knees keeping your back straight and knees apart. Like a man deep in thought.

STEP 2: BREATHE

Take a deep belly breath in. As you breathe out, gently tighten your abdominal muscles, if you need to push. Never hold your breath while pushing down. This creates an abnormal downward pressure on the pelvic floor muscles, which will cause them to tighten instead of relax. When this happens it's like trying to squeeze toothpaste out with the cap on. Eventually, prolonged straining and increased pelvic floor muscle tightness can result in hemorrhoids and pain during bowel movements. It could also exacerbate your overall pelvic pain.

STEP 3: GIVE YOURSELF TIME!

It's okay to sit on the throne for 15 minutes. Don't rush it. Rushing things might cause you to strain, maybe even feel 'not all the way done', which can also cause constipation, bloating or frequent unnecessary trips to the bathroom.

If having a bowel movement is painful, try applying an oil-based lubricant at the rectum to make the passage pain-free.

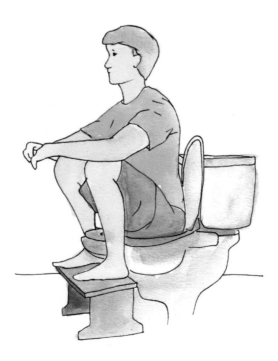

MINDFUL POOPING

Do you ever bring your iPhone, Kindle, or iPad into the bathroom with you? Come on, we're all guilty of it. And hands up who checks his email or uses this time to catch up on social media and whatnot?

Here's the thing, in a world full of distraction and stressors, it's easy for us to get sidetracked and lose ourselves in our devices. Despite what you might think, the brain isn't meant to multi-task. So says the research. The same part of the brain that decreases in size with persistent pain is found to do the same in those people who juggle lots of different apps, programs, games, etc. on their digital devices. These same structural changes are associated with anxiety and depression. And as you know, men with persistent pelvic pain also have high incidences of correlated depression and anxiety. So it's a double whammy.

Next time you bring your device to the bathroom for a number two, pay attention to what your body feels like. What do your shoulders and neck feel like? How's your breathing? Is it shallow or deep? Depending on what you're reading, playing or browsing, your body is most likely physically reacting to it, distracting your body from pooping.

A body under stress isn't going to have the urge to poop, remember? Ultimately, this will slow the process of digestion and elimination resulting in constipation.

IT'S 'GETTING HARD'

I know. All this talk about pelvic pain and poop is getting hard, maybe overwhelming. But that's not what I'm getting at here. I'm talking about boners. And exercising your right to pleasure yourself.

Sex and masturbation are good for you, but in moderation. Too much, and it could hinder your progress. During orgasm and ejaculation, your pelvic floor muscles contract strongly and tighten further above your baseline. Put simply, your pelvic floor muscles work harder, which can create more tension and pain afterwards. So if you're used to masturbating four or five times a day, maybe it's time to dial down a bit and 'prepare' for sex.

In practice, here's what I mean by that...

Don't make it robotic or pre-programmed.

Give yourself some time to feel your body, connecting with yourself and/ or your partner.

Give yourself some downtime afterwards so you can relax post-orgasm.

Be truthful with yourself.

Consider some of these factors... How do you feel during sex? How does your body feel during sex or masturbation? Are you calm or are you anxious? What are your pelvic floor muscles are doing? Are they tight or relaxed? What happens when you relax them? Are you rushing to masturbate because mom's knocking on the bathroom door yelling for you to come out? I kid, but situations like that truly do happen. You've probably experienced it yourself at one point in your life.

All these questions are geared towards bringing awareness back into your body, being able to accept yourself as a whole human being and not just a collection of body parts.

Phew! That's been some learning curve in the last two chapters. Everything from the brain, to sugar and cocaine, temper tantrums to pooping. Now that you've got a better understanding of the way your mind and body operate, let's go have some fun. It's time to put all of this into practice and start living a life without pain.

CHAPTER 6

THE NUTS AND BOLTS OF TREATING YOUR PELVIC PAIN

In this section of the book, I guide you through some practical, self-treatment techniques to help down-train your pelvic floor muscles to ease your pelvic pain. I want to preface this by saying these exercises aren't the be-all-and-end-all solution to your symptoms. No miracle cure. Every guy responds differently to treatment. I encourage you to take this information and play with it. Explore, be curious, and most importantly listen to your body. If you want to tweak some of the suggestions below, go for it! In fact, I want you to. These are just guidelines, not rules. The best treatments are those that you individualize and make your own. Remember, the goal is for you to be the expert in treating yourself.

BREATHE IN THE GOOD SH*T, BREATHE OUT THE BULLSH*T

Breathing is an essential part of life that most of us take for granted. As I mentioned already in earlier sections of the book, especially when talking about sleep, diaphragmatic breathing AKA belly breathing can be a game-changer. I've seen it benefit all my patients and I'm certain it will do the same for you too.

Typically, with stress and anxiety, your breathing patterns change to a shallower, faster type of chest breathing. Hmm, sorta sounds like the fight or flight scenario again. But it's okay. We're going to learn how to use breathing to turn the calming switch on.

First things first. Noticing what's happening right now. Go ahead and take a deep breath. Breathe in through your nose and out through your mouth.

What did you notice? What moved first? Belly or upper chest?

Try it again, paying attention to where you notice your breath the most.

Once you've taken a moment to witness what's normal for you, let's practice some diaphragmatic breathing and see how you go.

Find a comfortable sitting or lying-down position. At first, it might be easier to feel the fullness of the diaphragm and your breath while lying down.

Place your hands on the each side of your lower ribs. Settle in. Relax your shoulders, jaw and mouth. Gently close your eyes.

As you take a deep breath in, you should feel your belly and lower ribs rise upward and outward, sorta like a balloon. You should feel the back of your ribs gently expanding out towards the surface you're lying on.

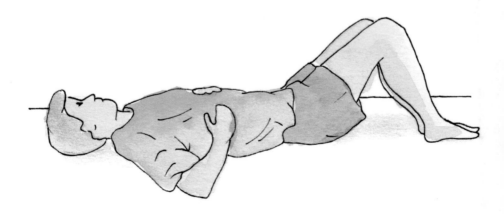

You might find yourself trying hard to focus on this breathing thing and it'll probably feel weird if you've never practiced this before. It's okay. You're learning, so cut yourself some slack if you don't get it right away. Accept what your body can do right now instead of forcing change. Forcing anything will create more resistance in your body, which defeats the purpose of letting go.

After you've practiced paying attention to your belly breathing pattern, let's add more awareness to your pelvic floor muscles.

PELVIC FLOOR RELAXATION USING YOUR BREATH

Get comfy. This would be a good time to invest in some pillows or even a bolster. Both will be helpful for this exercise.

When starting out, it's always useful to find a quiet space where you can focus on tuning into how your body's feeling. Connecting with the pelvic floor is no easy task, especially if all you know down there is pain.

With this exercise, we're going to explore sensations that you feel other than the pain. So I recommend gifting yourself 5-10 minutes of alone time. Maybe even pop on some relaxing music, if you're into that.

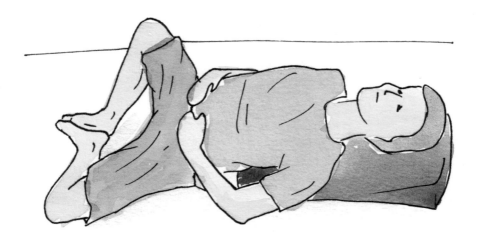

Start by sitting with your back facing the bolster or pillows. Slowly lower yourself down to rest your back on top of the bolster.

Bring your feet together so the soles of your feet touch, allowing your knees to open out to the side. If this posture is not comfortable for your back, feel free to try the same pose but without the bolster. If you feel like your legs are straining and inner thighs are too tight, use pillows for support underneath your knees.

This posture should feel comfortable. I love this restorative position because it opens the pelvic floor, and the feedback you get from your hands on your belly deepens the awareness of the belly and pelvic floor breathing.

As you take in your next breath, guide the breath into your lower ribs, belly and pelvic bowl. You should feel your belly soften as it expands, your sitz bones (the bony part of your butt that you sit on) separate, and the pelvic floor muscles lengthen out and down. You're doing it right if you feel the area between the base of your penis and anus bulge out slightly.

If you're still having a hard time feeling your pelvic floor muscles, place your hand between the area I just described to feel the subtle movement. As you breathe in, you should feel the pelvic floor muscle gently bulge, as if your tailbone is moving away from your pubic bone.

One more thing! Practice, practice, practice.

You don't just have to do it lying down on your back. Let this type of breathing keep you grounded throughout the day. Even when you think it's not working, keep trying because you're planting seeds for improvement.

Let go of instant gratification. Trust me, it gets easier the more you do it. The brain will eventually catch up and stop thinking you're in danger, allowing your muscles to let go. In the end, it will be automatic and ingrained in your brain so you won't have to think about it as much. To get there, you've got to retrain the brain and the body at the same time for optimal results.

LETTING GO AND ACCEPTING

This type of breathing works best when you can recognize and bring awareness to your triggers. Start to note when, what, and where you tend to hold tension in your body, paying special attention to your pelvic floor muscles. If you're tensing or gripping your butt throughout the day, most likely your pelvic floor muscles are doing the same. So use the breath to let go of the tension you feel at various times. This will help you take control of your body's reactions to various stressors.

For example, I had a patient tell me that he noticed his whole body tense up when he played video games. He would've never put two and two together until he started paying attention to how his body felt during certain activities and situations. Once he identified the trigger, he was able to train his muscles to stay relaxed while playing his favorite games.

Accepting and owning your pelvic pain is step one to healing yourself. There comes a time when you have to let go and stop worrying about it. It's easy to fall prey to acting like the victim and hating the world for cursing you with this nightmare. At the end of the day, you've got to realize that you're the boss. You're in control of this. Getting into the right state of mind is key. Some days are going to be easier than others, but the hope is that eventually you'll have fewer bad days and more good ones.

You're not alone. Finding a support system is important. This could be family, friends, support groups, journaling, counselors, meditation, therapists, furry pals, pretty much anything you want. Use this support system not only on those crummy days, but also on the good ones to help you celebrate all your progress.

A MIND FULL OF LESS

What do you think of meditation? Let me guess. 'It's not your thing', right? You don't have to be some Buddhist monk sitting cross-legged for hours on a mountaintop to get some peace of mind. In short, you don't have to be good at zen.

Practicing mindfulness is actually practicing a mind full of less. Less attention to doing, running around and focusing on your pain. It's taking a moment to breathe and take it all in. Dealing with pelvic pain is overwhelming with doctor visits, tests, scans, treatments, etc. Oftentimes, you lose yourself in the chaos of it all.

So what's mindfulness?

❯ Being in the moment
❯ Not doing
❯ Paying attention with purpose
❯ Re-directing your thoughts to what you're doing (from the current focus on pain)
❯ Training your brain to slow down
❯ Being in the moment without judging or trying to change anything
❯ Not being attached to the outcome
❯ Not practicing distraction

PRACTICING MINDFULNESS WITH PELVIC PAIN

Learning to be mindful during times of stress and pain can help maintain all your treatment efforts. Think about it. You work so hard at relaxing and letting go of your tension, but then throw yourself back into running around at 100 miles per hour like the Energizer Bunny. Quieting your nervous system throughout the day is vital.

When you first practice mindfulness, it's hard. I'm not here to lie to you. It'll take consistent practice to focus your attention on the present moment even if that moment is painful.

Be aware of the thoughts that go on in your head during times of pain but don't react to them. Don't be attached to the outcome or results. It's natural to want to react to pain by tensing up or distracting yourself, but I encourage you to not do that. Instead, I want you to recognize how your body's feeling and accept it without changing a thing. Sometimes you've got to 'go into something to get out of it.'

Remember when I said your thoughts change the way you feel? The same applies to the practice of mindful relaxation. Allow the thoughts to come in and out, but don't react to them. Stay neutral. The more you can integrate this practice in your daily life, the more control you're going to have over how you feel and how your body reacts to certain situations.

If you need help getting into the groove, try these apps:

- Headspace (headspace.com)
- Calm (calm.com)
- Insight Timer (insighttimer.com)
- Guided Mindfulness Meditation (mindfulnesscds.com) with mindfulness expert, Jon Kabat-Zinn, PhD
- Buddhify (buddhify.com)

Other mindful-like practices that you could try:

- Yoga – it's not just for chicks and Buddhist monks, bro. NFL players and the military have adopted yoga as part of their regular training routine. Go figure! Yoga helps reduce stress, pain, anxiety and improves flexibility, agility, and sexual health and function.
- Tai chi and Qigong – like yoga, these are centuries-old mind-body practices that involve mental focus and relaxation using certain movements, body postures and breathing. They can help reduce pain and stress while improving overall mood and quality of life.

> Dancing – oh yeah, shake it! Not only is it a good cardio workout, but you get all the feel-good benefits too. Go ahead, bust out that happy dance even if you're faking it.

On the subject of movement, let's continue on to some physical practices.

CHAPTER 7

LIMBER UP!

Stretching has many benefits on its own, but with these next exercises we're going to add in the practice of diaphragmatic or deep belly breathing that we learned in the last chapter to enhance your relaxation and heighten your body awareness.

With any new exercise regimen, there's a learning curve. Some days it might feel easier; other days you might just feel like the tin man. Not a problem, though. Trust your body and learn to listen to it. It's normal to feel some discomfort with stretching. Some patients tell me, 'It's a good kinda hurt.' But if it doesn't feel right, then back off. Maybe you need to modify your position or use props like pillows, blocks, or straps. The bottom line here is to tailor it to your body and specific needs. The 'no pain, no gain' concept doesn't apply, so don't try to be macho.

As far as a protocol or how many times you should be doing the moves, that's entirely up to you. I'm not one to tell you to stretch x number of times for x number of days. That's not how I work and neither does your body. I will tell you that those who get good results typically spend anywhere from one to two hours a day on self-care. In the beginning, this may seem like a lot and nearly impossible. Like, who has time for all that? But at the end of the day, it's all about priorities and this includes where you put yourself on that list. Are you going to need to do this for the rest of your life? Honestly, I don't know. You can't put a timeframe on healing. But just like your car, the maintenance light goes on every so often to remind you to change your oil. Well, the same applies to your body and self-care. Your body might gently nudge you here and there, when life's thrown you into the trenches. It's important to pick up on those subtle cues so that you can use all your tools and strategies to take care of yourself, instead of letting things snowball out of control. We all need to take care of our bodies. Health equals happiness so finding balance is optimal.

Side note: Quick stretches don't make any lasting structural changes to muscle length. It's kinda like a rubber band. If you just flick it once, the shape stays the same. But if you stretch it out and hold it for a longer length of time the rubber band actually gets looser. Keep that in mind throughout this section. 'Motion is lotion' and stretching is a great way to lubricate your muscles and juice up your nerves.

YOGI SQUAT

THIS IS A GREAT HIP STRETCH AND PELVIC FLOOR LENGTHENER.

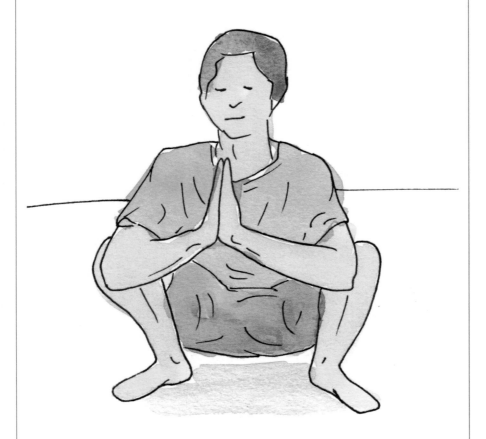

Start by standing with your feet wide apart and toes slightly pointed out to the side.

Slowly stick your butt out and lower yourself towards the floor. Keep your feet flat and your heels down. You shouldn't feel like you're holding yourself up.

🧍 **Take 5-10 deep breaths. As you breathe in you should feel a gentle bulging of your pelvic floor muscles and a widening of your sitz bones.**

🧍 **Stand up and repeat as needed.**

Finding that sweet spot will vary from person to person. If balance is an issue, feel free to lean your back up against a wall for added support. If your hips or knees just don't feel comfortable in this position, try adjusting the width of your knees and feet. I love props. Play around with a yoga block or pillow under your sitz bones. If you find your heels aren't touching the floor, use a rolled-up yoga mat or half foam roller under your heels.

THIS IS A GOOD ONE TO DO THROUGHOUT THE DAY.

COBRA POSTURE

THIS POSITION STRETCHES YOUR ABDOMEN, FRONT OF THE HIPS AND PELVIS.

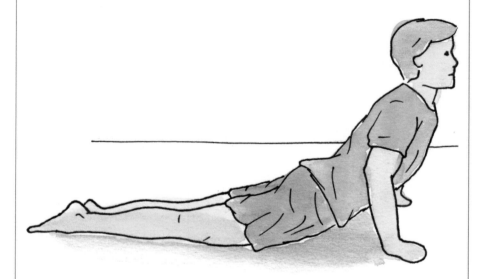

- Start by lying front down on your belly.

- Slide your elbows to your sides and roll your shoulders back and away from your ears. No ear-hugging with your shoulders! Keep your butt cheeks and legs soft throughout the entire stretch.

- Take a deep breath in as you prop yourself up onto your forearms.

- From here take 5 deep belly breaths.

If this doesn't feel like much of stretch, challenge yourself by straightening out your elbows all the way up (as shown in the picture). Again, keep your body as relaxed as possible as you hold the posture for an entire breath in and out.

Lower yourself slowly back down to your forearms.

Repeat 5 times or more if it feels right.

AIR SQUAT

THIS IS A GREAT HIP, LOW BACK AND PELVIC FLOOR STRETCH.

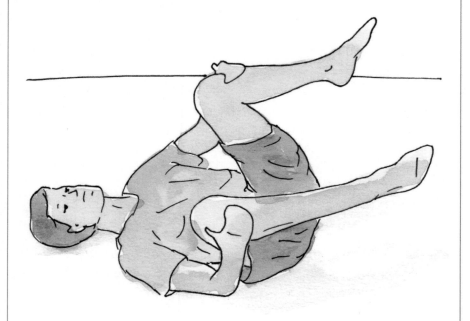

👦 Start by pulling both knees toward your chest.

👦 Take your knees out to the side to add in an inner groin stretch.

👦 As you're breathing, focus on letting go of your pelvic floor and buttock muscles with every breath in and keep them relaxed as you breath out. As you breathe in, you should feel a gentle bulging of your pelvic floor muscles and a widening of your sitz bones.

🧍 Take 5-10 deep belly breaths in this posture.

🧍 Repeat as needed.

If you find it hard to relax while keeping your knees up, rest your feet up on a wall for added support. With knees supported on the wall, you can enhance pelvic floor relaxation by doing some reverse Kegels.

REVERSE KEGELS

🧍 Take a full belly breath in. As you breathe out, gently let go of the tension around your anus as if you were trying to pass gas. You should feel a subtle bulge of your anus.

🧍 On your next breath out, focus on the front. The same technique applies but this time you're focusing on letting go of tension around the penis and testicles as if you were trying to pee.

Practice this technique several times, synchronizing it with your breath. Alternate between the front and the back. Never force or bear down while holding your breath. Big no-no!

LET'S TWIST

STRETCHING YOUR HIPS AND LOWER BACK HELPS TO REDUCE TENSION IN YOUR PELVIC FLOOR BECAUSE THEY SHARE THE SAME REGION AS THE PELVIS.

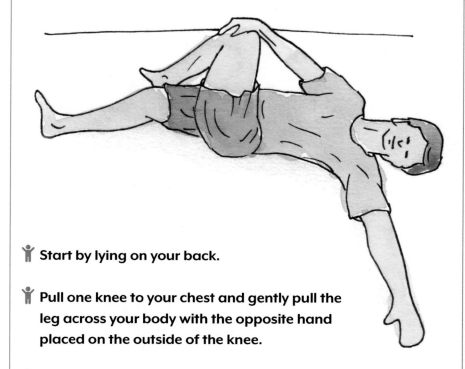

🧍 **Start by lying on your back.**

🧍 **Pull one knee to your chest and gently pull the leg across your body with the opposite hand placed on the outside of the knee.**

🧍 **Extend the other arm out to the side at shoulder level.**

🧍 **To increase the intensity of this stretch, turn your head to look at your extended arm.**

🧍 **Breathe deeply for 5-10 breaths.**

🧍 **Repeat on the other side. And remember, no butt-gripping!**

PIGEON STRETCH

The muscles of the hip connect intimately with the pelvic floor muscles, especially the obturator internus. This muscle originates inside the pelvis and attaches to the outside of your hip. The connective tissue of this muscle is shared by the pelvic floor muscles. An important nerve that innervates the pelvic floor muscles also runs across this muscle. So stretching the hips is essential.

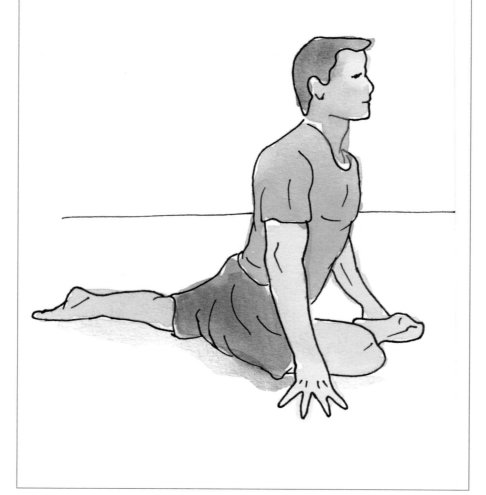

👤 Start on all fours.

👤 Slide one knee in between your hands. The knee should be closer to one hand and the foot towards the other hand, with the outer edge of the lower leg resting on the ground.

👤 Next straighten your other leg, resting the top of the knee and foot on the floor.

👤 If this is a deep enough stretch for you, stay here. If you're looking for a bit more, lower yourself down onto your forearms.

👤 If you're feeling like the kinda guy who can bend himself into any shape, lower yourself all the way by sliding your arms out straight in front of you.

👤 Remember to breathe and keep your butt, hips and pelvic floor muscles relaxed.

👤 Hold this stretch for at least a minute.

👤 Repeat on the other side.

SEATED FORWARD BEND

CAN YOU TOUCH YOUR TOES? IF YOUR HAMSTRINGS ARE ANYTHING LIKE MINE, BENDING FORWARD TO TOUCH YOUR TOES IS ALMOST IMPOSSIBLE. THAT'S WHY I LIKE TO USE A LITTLE HELP FROM A BOLSTER, PILLOW, BLOCK, OR CUSHION. WHATEVER YOU WANT TO PUT UNDER YOUR BUM IS FINE WITH ME.

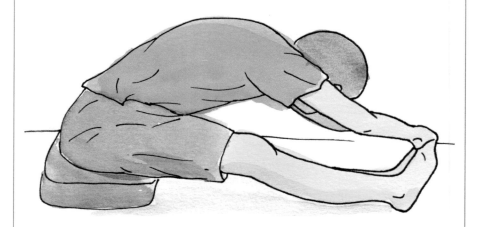

🧍 Start by sitting on the floor, legs straight out in front of you.

🧍 Slowly reach your hands forward, hinging at your hips with your back straight, until you feel a nice stretch in the back of your thighs and lower back.

🧍 Don't fret if you can't reach your toes and don't push it either. Just slide your hands as far down as possible and hold it there.

It could be as far as your thighs, below the knees or even shins. Adjust as needed and never force the stretch. A long strap could also be helpful here. If you're using a strap, sling it around the arches of your feet and use it as an anchor as you bend forward into the stretch.

🧍 Breathe deeply into your belly and the pelvis for several breaths. As you breathe in, you should feel a gentle bulging of your pelvic floor muscles and a widening of your sitz bones.

🧍 Feel the sitz bones gently separate with every breath in.

LUNGE

ALL THIS TALK ABOUT YOUR BACKSIDE, BUT WHAT ABOUT THE FRONT? THIS STRETCH IS USEFUL FOR STRETCHING THE FRONT OF THE HIP, GROIN, THIGH, AND ABDOMEN. IT'S HELPFUL TO DO THIS ONE ON A YOGA MAT OR SOFTER SURFACE.

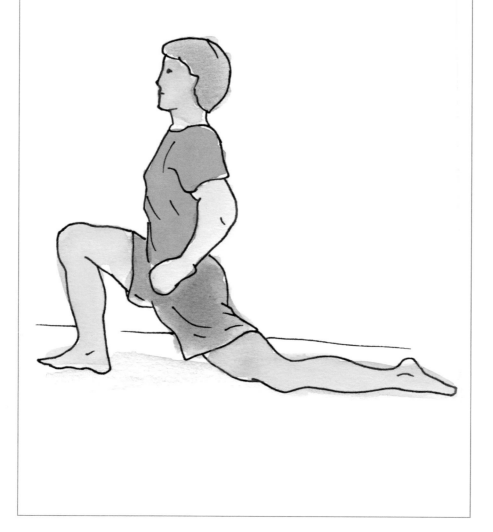

🧍 Start by kneeling on one leg with the other leg extended straight back, top of the foot resting on the floor.

🧍 Keeping your upper body nice and straight, lean forward shifting your weight onto the front leg. Be mindful not to have the knee go past the toes, as that would place excess strain on your knee. Feel free to explore rocking back and forth into the stretch, and even doing some small hip circles.

🧍 Hold for a minute then repeat on the other side. Listen to your tissues.

Do this one as many times throughout the day as you need.

MODIFIED THOMAS STRETCH

ANOTHER VARIATION OF THE LUNGE STRETCH IF THE KNEES AREN'T FEELIN' IT.

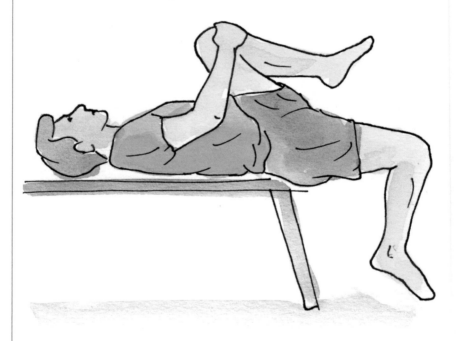

🧍 **Lie on a bench, edge of your bed, or anything sturdy that's off the ground. Key word: sturdy. Make sure it's high enough so your leg can dangle off the edge.**

🤸 **Bring one knee to your chest while the other dangles down. Let gravity gently do the stretching for you.**

🤸 **Make sure your back is relaxed and that you're breathing, noticing any tension and letting that tension go.**

Don't overthink it.

ADDUCTOR STRETCH

THIS STRETCH FOCUSES ON YOUR INNER GROIN MUSCLES, WHICH ATTACH TO YOUR PELVIC BONE AND CAN REFER PAIN TO THE PELVIC FLOOR.

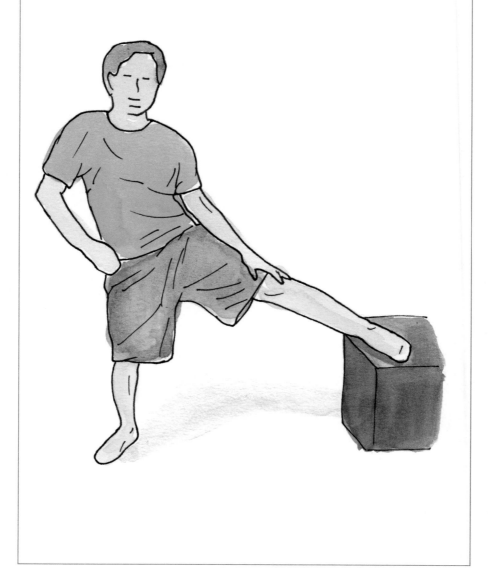

- ⅄ Find a step, curb, chair, pretty much anything you can confidently prop your leg on. Start with a small to medium step height.

- ⅄ Place one leg onto the step keeping the knee straight.

- ⅄ Slightly bend the knee on the standing leg to adjust the intensity of the stretch felt in your inner groin.

- ⅄ Keep your back straight and hips facing forward.

- ⅄ For better control of your hips, place your hands around your waist to stabilize your pelvis and hips keeping them from twisting.

- ⅄ If the stretch is too much for your knees or just uncomfortable, try propping your leg on a smaller step.

- ⅄ Hold this stretch for one minute and repeat on the other side.

- ⅄ Again, repeat as necessary.

MYOFASCIAL RELEASE

Fascia is what connects everything in the body. It's kinda like cellophane wrapping around organs, muscles, bones, ligaments, tendons, blood vessels, and nerves. You name it, if it's in the body, it's got fascia. And I hope I don't ruin food for you, but you know that white filmy stuff that you see when eating chicken off the bone? Yup, that's fascia!

Fascia has sensors that feed back information to the brain. Fascia used to be thought of as not really having an important role. Today, there's more research to support that fascia does in fact play a huge part in posture and body movement. Fascia is an interconnected 3D webbing throughout the whole body that provides structural support, disperses energy, and functions to allow for efficient and fluid movement.

The next couple of exercises come from Jill Stedronsky, MS, OTR and Brenda Pardy, OTR, in their book *Myofascial Stretching A Guide to Self-Treatment*[1]. I always recommend that patients get in the groove of myofascial stretching. It's one of the key components to balancing dysfunctions in the body and optimizing the environment for healing to take place.

You'll need two myofascial release balls[2]. I recommend using nothing bigger than 5 inches. Most balls come in 4 inches. You can go smaller but that will increase the intensity. Best to start off with 4-5 inches and experiment with other sizes once you get the hang of it.

SEEK AND DESTROY!

Here's the gist of what we're doing here with the myofascial release work. You're going to find spots on your body that aren't comfortable and work them out. Breathing is key to the release. Just like pelvic floor relaxation exercises, this also requires some mindful focus.

What you feel will vary from person to person. Some have described feelings of pulsing, tingling, heat, rug burn, deep stretch, throbbing or tightness. Having some sort of sensation while doing myofascial release work is normal. Some of the pain you feel might even be reproduced. Don't worry. If you can find it, you can treat it. Myofascial release can be uncomfortable so just listen to your body. If you need to back off, back off. You don't want to treat pain with more pain.

For all releases, you have to hang out for a bit. Generally one or two minutes in each spot. Could be less, could be more, depending on how your body feels. Remember all that deep belly breathing we practiced earlier? This would be a great place to use that skill.

FRONT OF THE HIP AND PELVIS

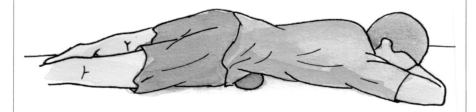

🧍 First, find the pelvic bone by placing your hands around your waist.

🧍 Next, slide your fingers in front of your hips to feel for the bony landmarks on either side. Then lie face down with one ball just inside the pelvic bone, just in the crease of your groin. Pull the opposite knee up towards your armpit, like a frog leg.

🧍 Breathe into the area of the ball allowing your pelvic floor muscles to relax and lengthen during the release. No butt-gripping!

ABDOMEN

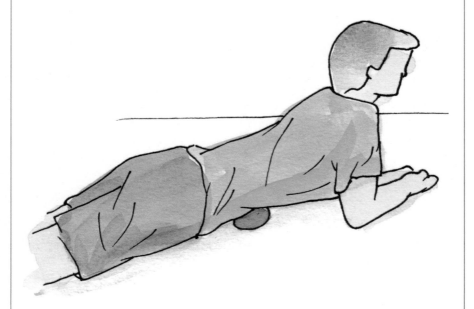

🕺 Start by lying on your stomach. Place the ball slightly above and off to one side of your belly button. Avoid placing the ball directly on top of the ribs. The ball is meant to be just underneath the ribs into soft tissue. Breathe, relax and allow your belly to melt over the ball like butter. Little by little, inch the ball down until you reach the pelvic bowl.

🕺 Along the way make sure to stop and release any tender points you may find.

🕺 You can prop yourself up onto your elbows to increase the stretch or you can choose to lay flat, resting your head into your forearms.

SPINE

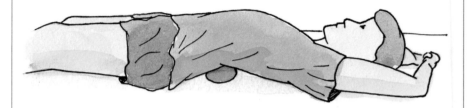

🧍 For this exercise, you can choose to use one ball down the middle of the spine or use two balls on either side of the spine. Choose the one that feels best to you.

🧍 Start at the base of the spine resting the ball directly underneath the sacrum (triangular bone at the end of the spine). Experiment with knees straight or bent, arms over the head or out to the side. Slowly work your way up the spine, one segment at a time.

🧍 Breathe and relax into each spot. Some spots may be more tender than others, requiring more attention.

LOWER BACK

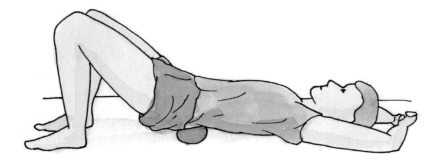

 Lie with two balls on either side of your lower back. Bend knees to add more pressure onto the balls.

 To address tender points in the deep back muscles, try pulling one knee up towards your chest. After the release, switch to do the other side.

 You can also put one ball directly on the sacrum, a triangular bone at the end of your spine, to release the pelvis.

 As always, use your breath to enhance the release and relax your pelvic floor muscles.

There are many more releases described in the Stedronsky Pardy book, but these are the ones I've found to be most helpful and effective in treating pelvic pain.

TRIGGER POINTS: WHAT, WHY AND HOW

Trigger points feel like tight bands of muscle fibers within a muscle, AKA a "muscle knot." They're a clinical phenomenon that leaves us clinicians scratching our heads. They're also referred to as 'tender points' depending on who you talk to. Personally, I like to call them tender points (sounds less scary if you ask me).

The best way to describe referred pain is using the heart attack example. When a heart attack is felt, the person will usually have a strong, painful sensation down the left arm. The brain gets a lot of information sent its way up the spinal cord. So it's getting info not only from your body but also the environment. Therefore, when the brain responds sending a signal back down to your body, it's taking a guess and sometimes this can lead to pain elsewhere in the body. In the heart attack analogy, the input coming up your spinal cord is not only from your heart but everything else that's feeding into the same neural pathway.

Don't forget that danger detectors like to sprout, expanding their curiosity to other parts of your body. It's like an annoying boss trying to micromanage every department underneath him.

Trigger points can be tricky to find in your own body, especially without the guidance of some trained hands. If you get stuck, I recommend getting in touch with a pelvic floor therapist to teach you how to find and treat them.

When it comes to what they feel like and how you might go about doing this for yourself, they can range in size from a grain of rice to as big as a chestnut or maybe even bigger. Trigger points feel like a 'muscle problem', lumpy and ropey. They can leave you feeling achy, stiff, dull, tired and heavy. No-one really knows why trigger points surface, but we all have the potential to experience them. It's worth noting that not everyone with trigger points has pain so we can't go pointing a finger at them just yet. Possible causes are stress, lack of nutrient-dense diet, direct injury, old injuries, postural stressors, lack of movement, overexertion and so forth. They also respond to psychological stress, which means these points get extra sensitive when you're stressing out.

There's a great workbook called *The Trigger Point Therapy Workbook*[3] by Clair and Amber Davies, NCBTMB, which goes into a lot more detail about trigger points and self-treatment. This workbook is based on copious research and work from the pioneers of trigger point release doctors Janet Travell and David Simons. Paul Ingraham also has an ebook tutorial about trigger points. You can get hold of it at www.painscience.com/tutorials/trigger-points.php. His style of writing is great, very tongue-in-cheek, and fun to read. For the purposes of this book, I'm going keep it simple.

HOW TO FIND AND MASSAGE TRIGGER POINTS

You know more than anyone else about what, where, and how much it hurts. So who better to treat it than you?! Of course, getting expert hands to guide you is ideal but learning how to apply these techniques to yourself is priceless.

Find the most sensitive areas that feel good to massage. If it feels like a pulse or gives you sharp shooting, radiating, burning pain, that's probably a blood vessel or nerve so back off!

Lots of my patients like to use tools to help them with trigger point massage. The myofascial balls you use for the myofascial release would be great to use to release trigger points. Something firmer that's also cheap is a good ol' fashioned tennis ball. You don't need anything fancy. A tennis ball is good for areas like the butt, inner and outer thigh; you know, the meatier muscles. If your points are extra sensitive, I'd recommend sticking with the myofascial ball, then progressing to something firmer like the tennis ball once pressure is tolerated. I also suggest using a massage stick[4] for the inner groin, outer thigh, hamstrings, calves, or whatever else feels good. I wouldn't recommend using a tennis ball on the abdomen. Use myofascial balls there instead. Or you can just use the best tool that money can't buy, your hands!

Get to know and feel your body. Initially, you probably won't be able to feel much, but as you fine-tune your skills, you'll be able to pick up on the more obvious.

When massaging, please please don't poke, prod, or hit yourself. Trust me, I've seen it all, otherwise I wouldn't be telling you this. Being too aggressive can backfire on you. Use gentle, stroking, kneading massage to feel your muscle tissue. Try hand-over-hand for added support, or make a fist supporting your thumb on your index finger, if you need to get at smaller or more specific areas.

HAND-OVER-HAND

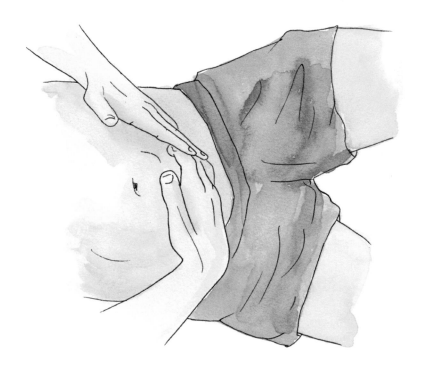

Be mindful of your pressure. Moderate pressure is okay. If you go too light, you might just be gliding your skin. So find that happy medium. On a scale of 1-10 with 10 being off-the-wall pain and discomfort, you want to be somewhere around 4-5. If you're flinching, guarding or tensing your muscles, it kinda defeats the purpose of the release.

SUPPORTED THUMB

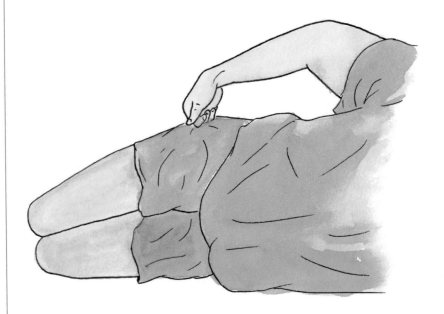

Use small stroking, circular, kneading or scooping motions during the release with whatever tool you wish to use. This can be in any direction. You can even put your whole body into it, like a rocking motion, or you can gently hold pressure over the point. To reduce some of the friction, use a dab of shea butter or massage cream.

How long you should treat the area all depends on you, your body's tissue tolerance, and the time you want to invest in treating yourself. Self-treatment can range anywhere from 30 seconds to 5 minutes. Of course, you could work longer. If it feels good, why not?

Let's keep it simple and start where it hurts.

Here are some common trigger points that are helpful to find on yourself:

ILIOPSOAS

A deep muscle that comes from your lower back attaching to the front of your pelvic bone. It sits behind your intestines and colon, and helps to flex your hip and back. Trigger points here can refer to the scrotum (nut sack), front of the thigh and abdomen. The myofascial ball abdomen release and soft tissue mobilization (discussed later on in the book) helps tackle these points well. You can use your hands to release this muscle but I would learn this from a licensed professional first before experimenting.

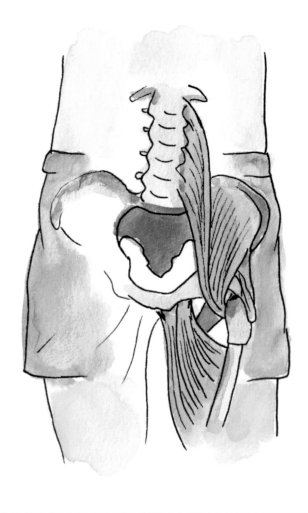

PAIN REFERRAL PATTERN OF ILIOPSOAS

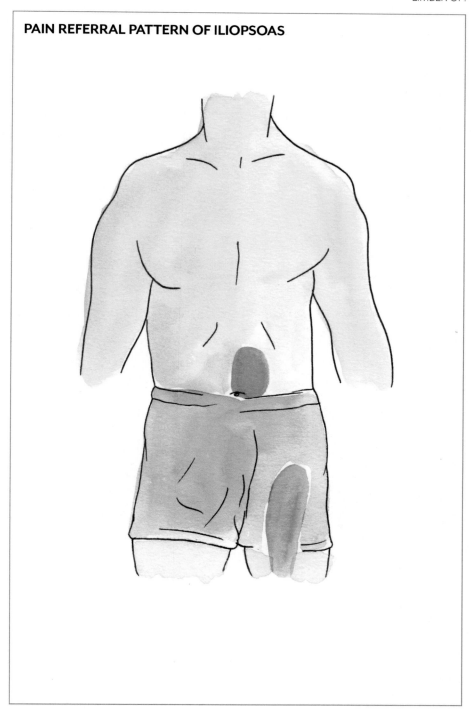

BULBOSPONGIOSUS AND ISCHIOCAVERNOSUS

These muscles make up part of the outermost layer of your pelvic floor. The bulbospongiosus is found at the base of the penis and the ischiocavernosus is found traveling from your sitz bones to the base and side of the penis. Trigger points here can send pain to the penis, anus, and perineum (area between anus and scrotum). Gently use your finger pads to find tender points and massage them away.

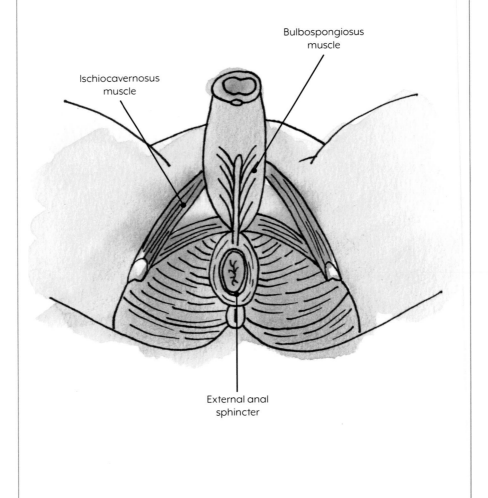

Bulbospongiosus
muscle

Ischiocavernosus
muscle

External anal
sphincter

GLUTEUS MAXIMUS

This is the big muscle that makes up the meaty part of your butt. It extends from your pelvic bone, sacrum and tailbone, and attaches to the top of the thigh bone, meshing with the connective tissue of the outer thigh, also known as the iliotibial tract or, as you might know it, the IT band.

Trigger points here can refer pain into the hip, butt, tailbone, or sacrum. Oftentimes, trigger points here can feel like a real deep 'pain in the ass.' Use a tennis or myofascial release ball to massage out trigger points here. Place the ball between you and the wall or sit or lie down on it for a more intense release.

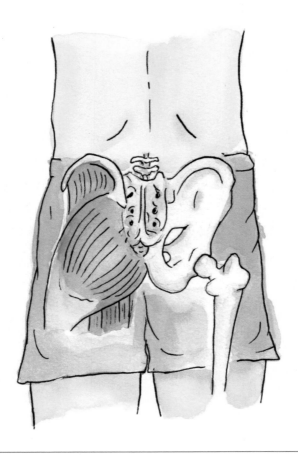

PAIN REFERRAL PATTERN FOR GLUTEUS MAXIMUS

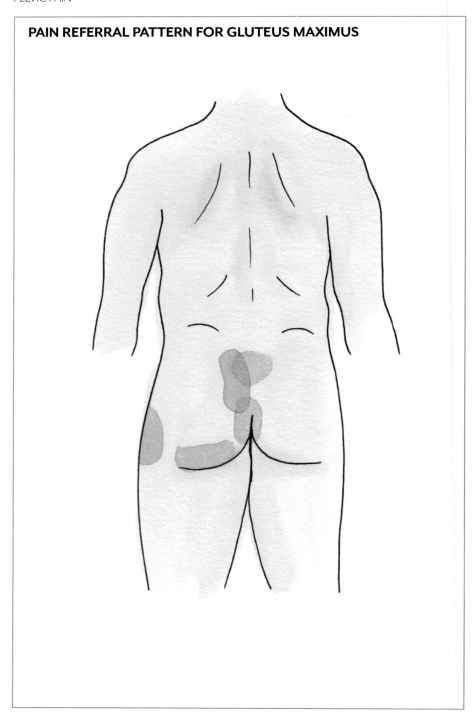

MYOFASCIAL BALL RELEASE TO GLUTEUS MAXIMUS

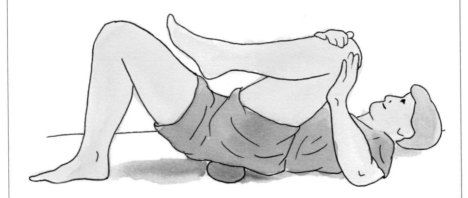

🧍 Lie on your back placing one myofascial ball underneath your butt cheek just a tad off toward the outside of your hip. Bend the knee on the same side up to your chest to give you more leverage and freer motion. While lying on the ball, move around to find the 'sweet spot.'

🧍 Experiment with circular, up-down or side-to-side rolling motions as you perform the release. You can choose to roll onto your side to tackle the outer hip muscle attachments as well.

🧍 Be cautious with putting the ball directly under your sitz bones as there are important nerves and blood vessels supplying your pelvic floor muscles that course through this region.

IT BAND FOAM ROLLING

TO RELEASE TRIGGER POINTS OF THE OUTER THIGH MUSCLE AND CONNECTIVE TISSUE, USE A FOAM ROLLER OR MYOFASCIAL BALL.

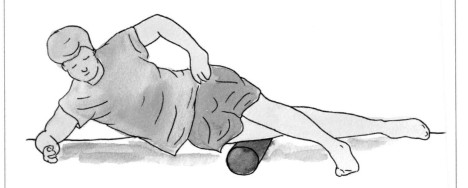

🧍 Start by lying on your side with the meaty part of your outer thigh on the foam roller. Bring the top leg out in front of you. Then use the foam roller to roll your bottom thigh from the top of your hip to just above your knee.

🧍 Make adjustments of your body weight on top of the foam roller based on your comfort level. This one can be a doozy, so start low and go carefully, listening to your body as you move along.

🧍 Repeat on the other side.

OBTURATOR INTERNUS

This muscle is found on the inside of the pelvic bowl and attaches to the outside of your hip bone. It helps to rotate your leg outward and extend your hip. Pain can be referred to the back of your thigh, butt, rectum, and you may experience feelings of fullness around the tailbone.

Here you can use the myofascial release or tennis balls just like you did for your glutes. Most often, massaging the glutes will address the outer part of the obturator internus. You can also access this muscle internally, which I'll go into later in the internal pelvic floor release section.

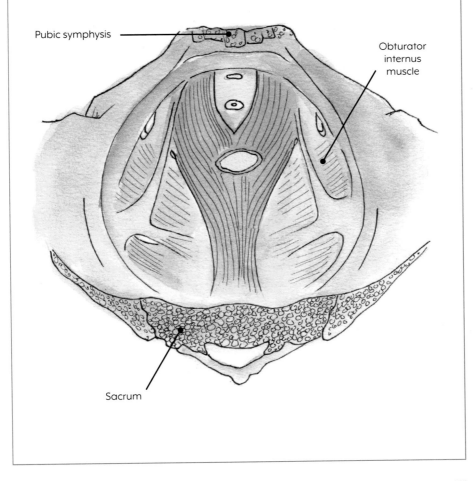

Pubic symphysis

Obturator internus muscle

Sacrum

ADDUCTOR MAGNUS

This muscle extends from the groin and the sitz bones to attach just above the inside of the knee. Trigger points here can refer pain to the inner groin, front of the thigh, inside of the pelvis, bladder, prostate, or rectum. You can use a massage stick to address trigger points here or just use your hands.

ADDUCTOR MAGNUS (BACK VIEW)

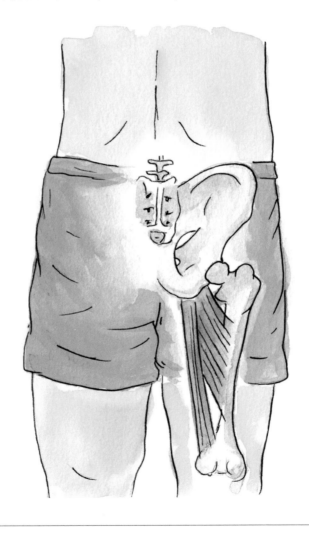

PAIN REFERRAL PATTERN FOR ADDUCTOR MAGNUS

ADDUCTOR MAGNUS RELEASE USING YOUR HANDS

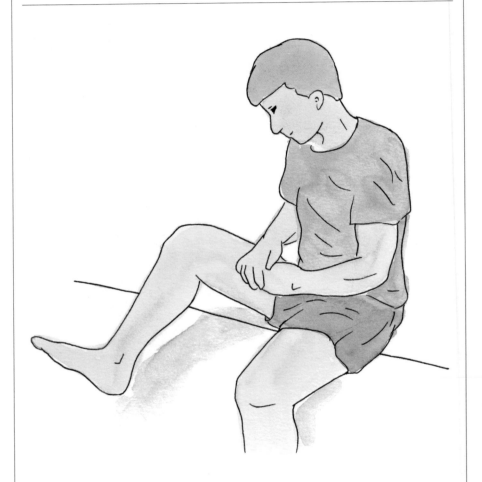

You can use the hand-over-hand technique to massage the muscle or use the supported thumb technique to release specific trigger points you find all along the adductor muscles.

PERINEAL MEMBRANE

The perineal membrane is a connective tissue layer found at the middle layer of the pelvic floor muscles and sits below the prostate. Trigger points here can refer pain to the base or tip of the penis, prostate, testicles, perineum or groin. To release this area, you can use two or three fingers to massage the area between the pubic bone and the base of the penis. When feeling for this area, it should feel like a trampoline, firm but elastic. If it's not so elastic, you've got some work to do. It's helpful to feel the other side as well to compare. To watch a video demonstrating the perineal membrane release go to drsusieg.com/book.

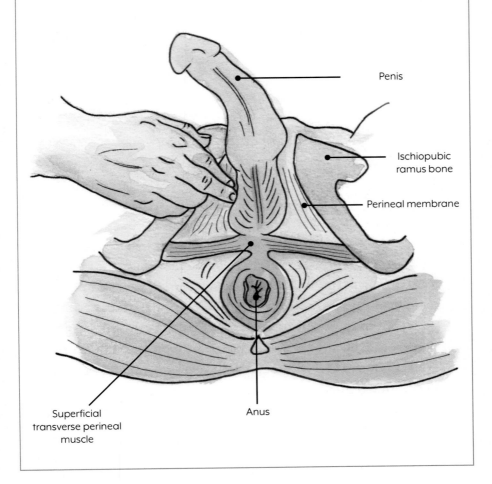

Penis

Ischiopubic ramus bone

Perineal membrane

Superficial transverse perineal muscle

Anus

CONNECTIVE TISSUE MANIPULATION AKA SKIN-ROLLING

Connective tissue manipulation is a technique I use to help loosen up connective tissue restrictions, promote increased blood flow and tissue health to soft tissue, and also stimulate the 'rest and digest' response mechanism of the nervous system. Skin-rolling is a technique that takes some time getting used to and practice to get it down pat. So be patient with this one.

It's easier to do this lying down with your back propped up on your headboard or somewhere semi-reclined, maybe your favorite recliner? It's done on bare skin and your fingernails need to be short. Trust me, you don't need nails digging into your skin.

Just like trigger point release, the technique itself can be a bit uncomfortable at first especially if you have restrictions. Use a dab of massage cream or shea butter, though not too much because you want to make sure you've got some traction and aren't just gliding all over the place.

🧍 **Start by picking a spot on your belly to practice. Place your thumbs together so that the thumbnails are touching each other. Place them on your skin and gently push in about 25%, so not a lot of pressure. Then take the rest of your fingertips and put them about 2 or 3 inches in front of your thumbs or wherever they lie naturally.**

🧍 **Roll your thumbs through the tissue as you simultaneously gather and lift the tissue up and away with your fingertips. You can move in any direction as you're rolling. This is a tricky technique and is best learned from an experienced therapist. To access the video on connective tissue manipulation, go to drsusieg.com/book.**

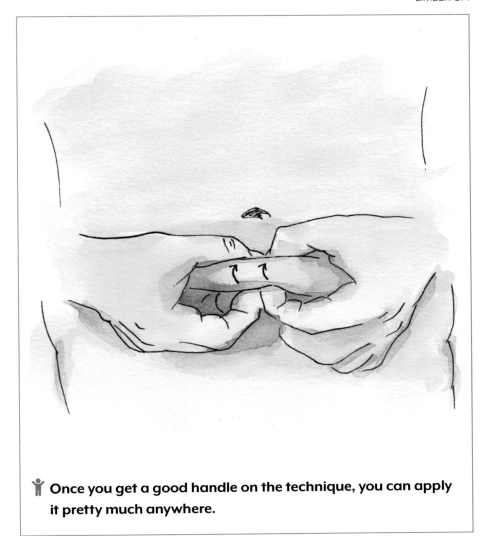

🤸 Once you get a good handle on the technique, you can apply it pretty much anywhere.

Here are some areas of connective tissue tension and tender points commonly found:

- ❯ Abdomen
- ❯ Just above your pubic bone, area around bladder
- ❯ Inner groin
- ❯ Inner thighs
- ❯ Inner glutes
- ❯ Top of the thigh

It's normal to feel some discomfort and have redness after doing trigger point or skin rolling techniques but don't go overboard. You can also experience some bruising if you tend to bruise easily. You might be sore too, but this typically doesn't last long. It's a bit like after you have a tough workout and your muscles are sore the next day. Remember we're not treating pain with pain. We're creating safety in your body so go easy on yourself and dose your treatment appropriately. You might be sore but you're safe. No harm is being done.

SOFT TISSUE MOBILIZATION FOR THE ABDOMEN

I teach patients how to mobilize their own fascia and connective tissue on their abdomen and just above their pubic bone. This helps release any restrictions in the fascia and soft tissue associated with pelvic floor restrictions. It will also address iliopsoas tension. I like to use the scoop and swoop technique.

🧍 **Start by lying down on your back with your knees bent up, or supported by pillows or a bolster.**

🧍 **Overlap your fingers as wide or as narrow as you'd like depending on the area you're treating.**

👱 Gently sink inside the part of your lower belly where the bony part of your pelvis sticks out. You should be able to make a half moon shape with your hands.

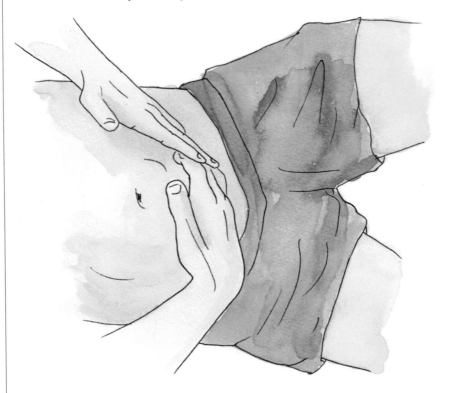

👱 Sink in scooping and swooping up as you massage up towards your belly button.

This technique can be done in all directions and anywhere on your abdomen or inner thigh.

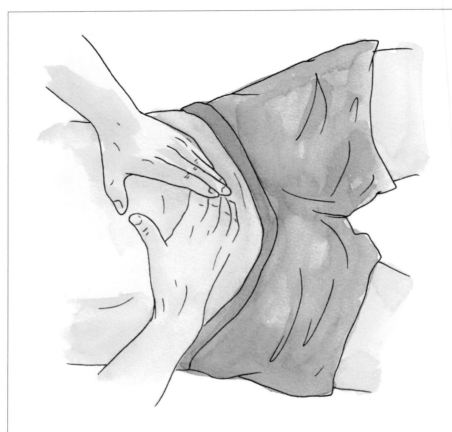

Since this is also kinda tricky to get a grasp on through words, I've made a video for you to follow at drsusieg.com/book.

If you're sore for several days or it really flares up, you may have been too aggressive and need to go a lighter next time. I've said it before, but I'll say it again. Always listen to your body and never push it past your limit. Recognize what those limits are and be comfortable with them. You'll get better results that way without the risk of a flare-up.

And if you need some expert hands to further guide you, get in touch with a pelvic floor therapist who can help.

INTERNAL PELVIC FLOOR RELEASE

Just because you can't see them doesn't mean your pelvic floor muscles don't get tight or have tender points. Internal pelvic floor muscle release is an important part of managing your pelvic pain symptoms. For internal releases, you can choose to use your middle or index finger, or use what I like to call an extension of my finger, the TheraWand©[5].

The TheraWand© was created with input from physical therapists to help patients treat their own pelvic floor muscles internally. I like the LA-Wand version because it's smaller in diameter which is great for pelvic floor muscle releases. It also has a naturally curved design to make trigger point release comfortable for both your hands, body, and pelvic floor muscles. To access the video on internal pelvic floor release go to drsusieg.com/book.

SO HOW DO YOU USE IT?

Here's what you'll need to get started:

- An open mind
- An organic water-based or oil-based lubricant[6]
- Two to four pillows
- Time
- Privacy
- TheraWand©
- A towel for clean up
- Relaxing meditation music (optional)

Follow these steps to perform the release:

1. Wash your hands.
2. Start by getting yourself comfortable. Prop yourself up in bed and use plenty of pillows so your back is supported.

3. You can bend your knees. I like to recommend supporting the outer knees with pillows so you don't have to strain keeping them up.
4. Apply generous amounts of lubricant to the tapered end of the wand.

ILLUSTRATION TO ACCOMPANY POINT 7

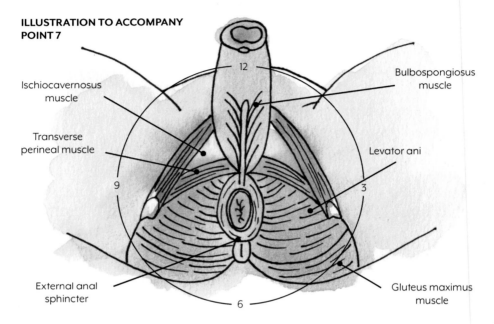

Ischiocavernosus muscle

Transverse perineal muscle

External anal sphincter

Bulbospongiosus muscle

Levator ani

Gluteus maximus muscle

12

9

3

6

5. Gently lift your penis and testicles up and out of the way.
6. Find your anus. If you need help, use a mirror.
7. Orient yourself to the anal opening like a clock, 12 o'clock being your pubic bone (in front), and 6 o'clock, your anal opening.
8. Gently, slowly insert the tip of the wand into the anal opening, which is at 6 o'clock. Take a few moments to breathe here. If there's some discomfort or difficulty inserting the wand, try to gently tighten your pelvic floor muscles and let go. Do this a few times. Once it's comfortable to insert the wand about one knuckle length in, hold it there and take a few deep belly breaths.
9. As you breathe in and out, feel the expansion and lengthening of your pelvic floor muscles. You should feel your anus opening and slightly bulging with every in-breath. You can do this for 1, 5, or even 10 minutes – whatever feels right for you at that time.

ILLUSTRATION TO ACCOMPANY POINT 10

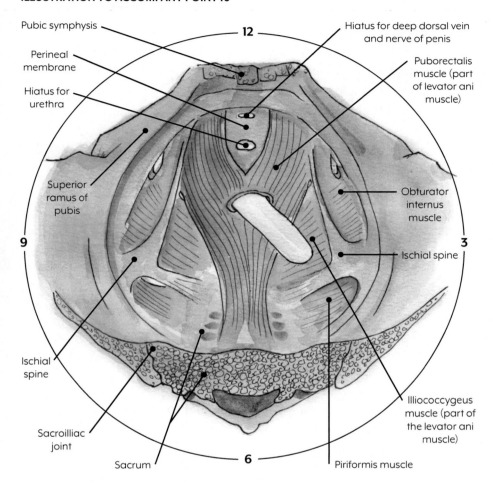

Pubic symphysis

12

Hiatus for deep dorsal vein and nerve of penis

Perineal membrane

Puborectalis muscle (part of levator ani muscle)

Hiatus for urethra

Superior ramus of pubis

Obturator internus muscle

9

3

Ischial spine

Ischial spine

Illiococcygeus muscle (part of the levator ani muscle)

Sacroilliac joint

Sacrum

6

Piriformis muscle

10. If you feel comfortable to continue, move the wand inward so that you're in about two to three knuckle lengths deep in total. Do not go past the first curve of the wand. From here, gently, slowly, sweep the wand by bringing the handle away from you and to the left, positioning the inserted tip from 6 o'clock to 11 o'clock. Return to the 6 o'clock starting position and sweep the wand by bringing the handle away from you and to the right, positioning the inserted tip from 6 o'clock to 1 o'clock. Avoid direct pressure at 12 o'clock, because your prostate and other important structures sit just behind the pubic bone.

11. While sweeping, see if you can find any tender spots. If you do, feel free to apply gentle pressure to the area and hold while you simultaneously guide your breath to that area. Hold for 90 seconds. Again the pressure you apply should not be agonizing. It can be uncomfortable but tolerable.

12. Anal tissue can be sensitive and at first might make you feel like you 'gotta go' or it might feel like a lot of pressure. Don't be alarmed. It's normal. Use deep breathing to help let go of the tension you feel. If sweeping is too uncomfortable, just move the wand to get to the next clock region. For example, go from 6 o'clock to 8 o'clock.

13. As an alternative, you can choose to use your own finger to give you better feedback and precision for finding trigger points. You would

ILLUSTRATION TO ACCOMPANY POINT 14

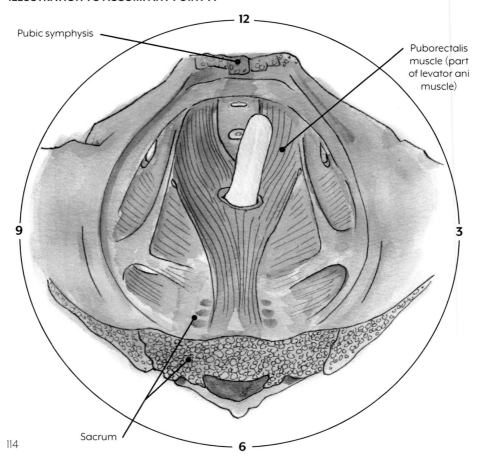

use your finger in the same way, visualizing the clock and moving to each number on the face of that clock.

14. If you have pain at the tip of the penis or fullness in the prostate, look for tender spots in the puborectalis muscle at 11 o'clock and 1 o'clock, just behind the pubic bone.

15. Obturator internus tender points can cause rectal pain or fullness, pain in the perineum, tailbone pain, hip pain or pain in the back of the thigh. To access the obturator internus muscle, direct the wand or your finger about 90 degrees from the 6 o'clock position so it's actually turned towards 3 o'clock or 9 o'clock on the other side. At this point, the wand should be about two knuckle lengths deep.

ILLUSTRATION TO ACCOMPANY POINT 15

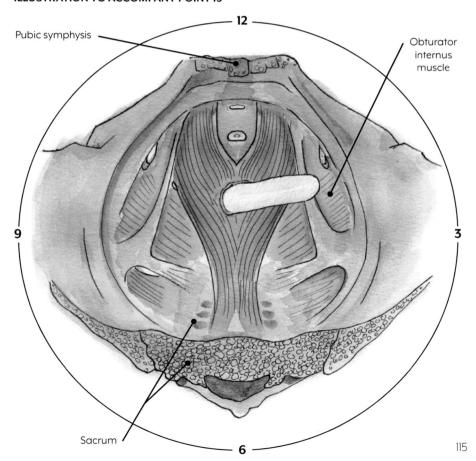

16. Always use caution, listening to your body and tissues. It's wise to consult with a physical therapist prior to use.

1–6   You can find this product through the resources section on my website at drsusieg.com/resources. Please note this is an affiliate product – see disclosure statement.

CHAPTER 8

DON'T GIVE UP!

While there's so much more I'd love to write about and teach you, this is not a textbook. Your body is unique. Treating it doesn't stop here at the page. What I've shared with you will guide you in the right direction and give you support on your healing journey. Who knows? Maybe you even had a good laugh here and there! (Humor me please!)

Every person responds differently to treatment so I can't guarantee how you're going to feel, but if you trust in your body, everything else will fall into place. Sometimes fear is what binds us from truly being free. So the next time you think, 'This is never going to go away,' ask yourself, 'What if the opposite were true?'

WHEN THE GOING GETS TOUGH, FIND THE RIGHT BUFFS

Ever heard of the African proverb, 'It takes a village to raise a child'? Well, the same goes for persistent pelvic pain. It takes a team of wellness practitioners to support you throughout your journey, so never feel like you have to go through this alone.

Wellness practitioners worth having by your side include:

- Pelvic floor therapist
- Integrative or functional medicine doctors
- Urologist

❯ Health coach
❯ Massage therapist
❯ Acupuncturist
❯ Nutritionist
❯ Psychologist
❯ Sex therapist

Of course, this isn't an exhaustive list, just some common wellness practitioners that I often consult with for my patients. It's worth saying that we're not all created equal. Just because you had a so-so experience with one practitioner doesn't mean that the next one will be just like him or her. So don't be afraid to get multiple opinions or consultations. Trust your gut. You need to find the best team that suits your needs and most importantly that is focused on working with you; not just telling you what to do. You bring your own unique strengths and resources to healing yourself. No-one is going to 'fix' you, because you're not broken.

Do you know when the healing really starts? When you can tell your story the way you want it to be heard.

PATIENCE IS GOLDEN

Persistent pelvic pain requires courage, effort, patience, and lots of TLC to tackle the good, the bad and the ugly that comes with it.

KNOW THAT YOU CAN LIVE A LIFE WITHOUT PAIN.

You might not be able to stop pain from knocking at your door but you certainly have the choice to not suffer. Don't let pain define your world. I'm sure there's a whole helluva lot more you'd like to be doing. So get up, get moving, and keep on keepin' on.

WHAT'S NEXT?

That said, if you've read this far and practiced the techniques but do need more help, don't be afraid to come find it! We all need to do some troubleshooting from time to time.

Questions might arise... 'What am I supposed to be feeling?', 'I put my hand where?', and 'I don't know if I'm doing this right.' These questions are common.

If you're anything like me, maybe you learn by doing and need a personal teacher guiding you through the steps. That more one-on-one attention is so helpful, which is why I created something special for you.

In my 6 Day Hands-On Training Program, you'll work one-on-one with me learning how to be the expert in treating yourself. You'll practice all the concepts and self-care techniques discussed in the book in addition to gaining boatloads of knowledge from picking my brain as we work together, access to all my professional networks and resources, and most importantly my undivided attention and support. Learn more at drsusieg. com/hands-on-training-program.

If you're ready to take matters into your own hands (no pun intended!) then connect with me at drsusieg.com to become the boss of your own health.

In loving wellness for your pelvis,

Dr. Susie Gronski, DPT, PRPC, WCS

BONUS!

As an extra gift for you, I've added some healthy, protein-packed smoothie recipes giving you a lil' food-as-medicine boost. Why use synthetic protein when you've got the real stuff? Don't worry about having mad skills in the kitchen, all you need is a blender. Phew!

ALMOND, PAPAYA AND DATE SHAKE

4 pitted and chopped dates

2 cups hemp milk

½ cup papaya

¼ cup raw cashews

5 ice cubes

1 tablespoon maple syrup
        or raw honey

Blend in high speed blender until smooth.

Makes 2 servings.

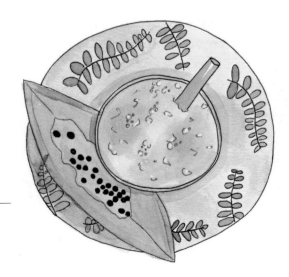

BRAZIL NUT CHERRY SMOOTHIE

1½ cups almond milk
¼ cup brazil nuts
1 tablespoon honey
2 cups pitted cherries
¼ teaspoon cinnamon
6 ice cubes

Blend in high speed blender
until smooth.

Makes 2 servings.

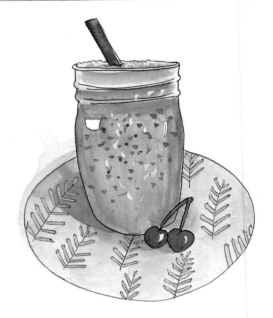

HEMP, RASPBERRY AND COCONUT SHAKE

2½ cups raspberries
1 cup apple juice
1½ cups canned coconut milk
4 tablespoons hemp seed
5 ice cubes
½ cup Greek or dairy-free yogurt

Blend in high speed blender
until smooth.

Makes 2 servings.

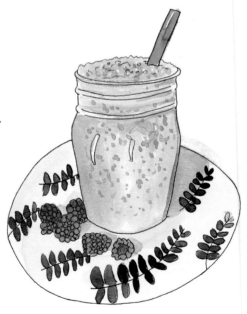

CHIA PIÑA COLADA

2 cups fresh pineapple choppe
1 cup coconut milk
2 tablespoons chia seeds
5 ice cubes
¼ cup raw sunflower seed
1 tablespoon raw honey

Blend in high speed blender until smooth.

Makes 2 servings.

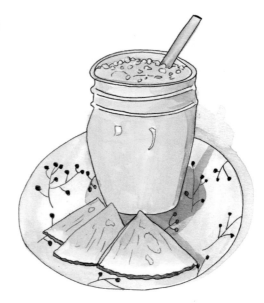

CANTALOUPE SURPRISE

½ teaspoon ground cardamon
1½ cups hemp milk
½ cantaloupe (seeded, peeled and chopped)
1 tablespoon honey
¼ cup raw almonds
¼ cup raw pumpkin seeds
5 ice cubes

Blend in high speed blender until smooth.

Makes 2 servings.

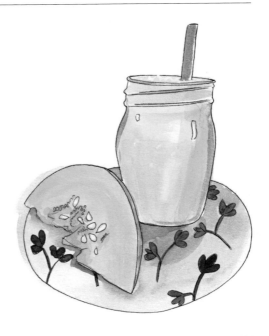

REFERENCES

Don't worry, I didn't make this up. But if you want to nerd out and read some dry, medical journal articles, then knock yourself out. Below are the references. Enjoy!

Pitts, M., Ferris, J., Smith, A., Shelley, J., Richters, J. (2008). Prevalence and correlates of three types of pelvic pain in a nationally representative sample of Australian Men. *The Journal of Sexual Medicine*, 5, 1223-1229.

Lin, P.H., Freedland, S.J. (2015). Lifestyle and lower urinary tract symptoms: what is the correlation in men? *Current Opinion in Urology*, 25, 1-5.

Faubion, S.S., Shuster, L.T., Bharucha A.E. (2012). Recognition and management of nonrelaxing pelvic floor dysfunction. *Mayo Clinic Proceedings*, 87(2), 187-193.

Shoskes, D.A., Nickel, J.C., Wagenlehner F.M.E. (2013). Management of chronic prostatitis/chronic pelvic pain syndrome (CP/CPPS): the studies, the evidence, and the impact. *World Journal of Urology*, 31(4), 747-53.

Shoskes, D.A., Berger, R., Elmi, A., Landis, J.R., Propert, K.J., Zeitlin, S. (2008). Adult urology: Muscle tenderness in men with chronic prostatitis/chronic pelvic pain syndrome: The chronic prostatitis cohort study. *The Journal of Urology*, 179(2), 556-560.

Nickel C., Shoskes D., Wang, Y., Alexander R.B., Fowler, J.E., Zeitlin S., O'Leary, M.P., Pontari, M.A., Schaeffer, A.J., Landis, R., Nyberg, L., Kusek, J.W., Propert, K.J., and the Chronic Prostatitis Collaborative Research Network Study Group. (2006). How does the pre-massage and post-massage 2-glass test compare to the Meares-Stamey 4-glass test in men with chronic prostatitis/chronic pelvic pain syndrome? *The Journal of Urology*, 176(1), 119-24.

Alexander, R.B., Propert, K.J., Schaeffer, A.J., Landis, R. Nickel, C., O'Leary, M.P., Pontari, M.A., McNaughton-Collins, M., Shoskes, D.A., Comiter, C.V., Datta, N.S., Fowler, J.E., Nadler, R.B., Zeitlin, S.I., Knauss, J.S., Wang, Y., Nyberg, L.M., Litwin, M.S., and the Chronic Prostatitis Collaborative Research Network Study Group. (2004). Ciprofloxacin or tamsulosin in men with chronic prostatitis/chronic pelvic pain syndrome. *Annals of Internal Medicine*, 141, 581-589.

Weidner, W., Anderson, R.U. (2008). Evaluation of acute and chronic bacterial prostatitis and diagnostic management of chronic prostatitis/chronic pelvic pain syndrome with special reference to infection/inflammation. *International Journal of Antimicrobial Agents*, 31S, S91-S95.

Tripp, D.A., Nickel, C.J., Wang, Y., Alexander, R.B., Propert, K.J., Schaeffer, A.J., Landis, R., O'Leary, M.P., Pontari, M.A., McNaughton-Collins, M., Shoskes, D.A., Comiter, C.V., Datta, N.S., Fowler, J.E., Nadler, R.B., Zeitlin, S.I., Knauss, J.S., Nyberg, L.M., Litwin, M.S., and the Chronic Prostatitis Collaborative Research Network Study Group. (2006). Catastrophizing and pain-contingent rest predict patient adjustment in men with chronic prostatitis/chronic pelvic pain syndrome. *The Journal of Pain*, 7(10), 697-708.

Chung, S., Lin, H. (2013). Association between chronic prostatitis/chronic pelvic pain syndrome and anxiety disorder: a population-based study. *PLOS ONE*, 8(5), e64630. doi:10.1371/journal.pone.0064630.

Nickel, C.J., Mullins, C., Tripp, D.A. (2008). Development of an evidence-based cognitive behavioral program for men with chronic prostatitis/chronic pelvic pain syndrome. *World Journal of Urology*, 26, 167-172.

Collins, M.M. (2003). The impact of chronic prostatitis/chronic pelvic pain syndrome on patients. *World Journal of Urology*, 21, 86-89.

Tan, H.M., Tong, S.F., Ho, C.C.K. (2012). Men's health: sexual dysfunction, physical, and psychological health—Is there a link? *The Journal of Sexual Medicine*, 9, 663-671.

Shoskes, D.A. (2012). Challenge of erectile dysfunction in the man with chronic prostatitis/chronic pelvic pain syndrome. *Current Urlology Reports*, 13, 263-267.

Wise, D.T., & Anderson, R.U. (2014). *A Headache in the Pelvis: A new understanding and treatment for chronic pelvic pain syndromes*. Occidental, CA: National Center for Pelvic Pain Research.

Naliboff, B.D., Stephens, A.J., Afari, N., Lai H., Krieger, J.N., Hong, B., Lutgendorf, S., Strachan, E., Williams, D. (2015). Widespread psychosocial difficulties in men and women with urologic chronic pelvic pain syndromes (UCPPS): case-control findings from the MAPP research network. *Urology*, 85(6), 1219-1327.

Kwon, J.K., Chang, I.H. (2013). Pain, catastrophizing, and depression in chronic prostatitis/chronic pelvic pain syndrome. *International Neurourology Journal*, 17, 48-58.

Jensen, M.P., Gianas, A., Sherliin, L.H, & Howe, J.D. (2015). Pain Catastrophizing and EEG- Asymmetry. *The Clinical Journal of Pain*, 31(10), 852-8. doi:10.1097/AJP.0000000000000182.

Strick, P.L., & Levinthal, D.J. (2012). The motor cortex communicates with the kidney. *Journal of Neuroscience*, 32(19) 6726-6731. doi: http://dx.doi.org/10.1523/JNEUROSCI.0406-12.2012.

Vandyken, C., Hilton, S. (2016). Physical therapy in the treatment of central pain mechanisms for female sexual pain. *Sexual Medicine Reviews*, 1-11.

Anderson, R.U., Sawyer, T., Wise, D., Morey, A., & Nathanson, B.H. (2009). Painful myofascial trigger points and pain sites in men with chronic prostatitis/chronic pelvic pain syndrome. *The Journal of Urology*, 182, 2753-2758.

Anderson, R.U., Wise, D., Sawyer, T., & Chan, C.A. (2006). Sexual dysfunction in men with chronic prostatitis/chronic pelvic pain syndrome: improvement after trigger point release and paradoxical relaxation training. *The Journal of Urology*, 176, 1534-1539.

Riegel, B., Bruenahl, C.A., Ahyai, S., Bingel, U., Fisch, M., Lowe, B. (2014). Assessing psychological factors, social aspects and psychiatric co-morbidity associated with chronic prostatitis/chronic pelvic pain syndrome in men—a systematic review. *Journal of Psychosomatic Research*, 77, 333-350.

Farmer, M.A., Chanda, M.L., Parks, E.L., Baliki, M.N, Apkarian, A.V., Schaeffer, A.J. (2011). Brain functional and anatomical changes in chronic prostatitis/chronic pelvic pain syndrome. *The Journal of Urology*, 186, 117-124.

Woodworth D., Mayer, E., Leu, K., Ashe-McNalley, C., Naliboff, D., Labus, J.S., Tillisch, K., Kutch, J.J., Farmer, M.A., Apkarian, A.V., Johnson, K.A., Mackey, S.C., Ness, T.J., Landis, R.J., Deutsch, G., Harris, R.E., Clauw, D.J., Mullins, C., Ellingson, B.M., MAPP Research Network. (2015). Unique microstructural changes in the brain associated with urological chronic pelvic pain syndrome (UCPPS) revealed by diffusion tensor MRI, super-resolution track density imaging, and statistical parameter mapping: A MAPP network neuroimaging study. *PLoS ONE*, 10(10): e0140250. doi:10.1371/journal.pone.0140250.

Kessler, T.M. (2016). Chronic pelvic pain syndrome: light at the end of the tunnel? *European Urology*, 69, 298-299.

Loh, K.K., Kanai, R. (2014). Higher media multi-tasking activity is associated with smaller gray-matter density in the anterior cingulate cortex. *PLOS ONE*, 9(9): e106698. doi:10.1371/journal.pone.010698.

Bordoni, B., Zanier, E. (2013). Anatomic connections of the diaphragm: influence of respiration on the body system. *Journal of Multidisciplinary Healthcare*, 6, 281-291.

Bordoni, B., Marelli, F., Bordoni, G. (2016). A review of analgesic and emotive breathing a multidisciplinary approach. *Journal of Multidisciplinary Healthcare*, 6, 97-102.

Park, H., Han, D. (2015). The effect of the correlation between the contraction of the pelvic floor muscles and diaphragmatic motion during breathing. *Journal of Physical Therapy Science*, 27, 2113-2115.

Anderson, R.U., Wise, D., Sawyer, T., Glowe, P., Orenberg, E. (2011). 6-day intensive treatment protocol for refractory chronic prostatitis/chronic pelvic pain syndrome using myofascial release and paradoxical relaxation training. *The Journal of Urology*, 185, 1294-1299.

Herati, A.S., Moldwin, R.M. (2013). Alternative therapies in the management of chronic prostatitis/chronic pelvic pain syndrome. *World Journal of Urology*, 4, 761-6.

Van Alstyne, L.S., Harrington, K.L., Haskvitz, E.M. (2010). Physical therapist management of chronic prostatitis/chronic pelvic pain syndrome. *Physical Therapy*, 90(12), 1795-1806.

Rosenbaum, T.Y., Owens, A. (2008). The role of pelvic floor physical therapy in the treatment of pelvic and genital pain-related sexual dysfunction. *The Journal of Sexual Medicine*, 5, 513-523.

Rosenbaum, T.Y. (2007). Pelvic floor involvement in male and female sexual dysfunction and the role of pelvic floor rehabilitation in treatment: a literature review. *The Journal of Sexual Medicine*, 4, 4-13.

Cohen, D., Gonzalez, J., Goldstein, I. (2016). The role of pelvic floor muscles in male sexual dysfunction and pelvic pain. *Sexual Medicine Reviews*, 4, 53-62.

Geneen, L.J., Martin, D. J., Adams, N., Clarke, C., Dunbar, M., Jones, D., McNamee, P., Schofield, P., Smith, B.H. (2015). Effects of education to facilitate knowledge about chronic pain for adults: a systematic review with meta-analysis. *Systematic Reviews*, 4, 132. doi: 10.1186/s13643-015-0120-5.

Butler D., and Moseley, L. (2014). *Explain Pain*. Australia. Noigroup Publications.

Lee, J.H., Lee, S.W. (2015). Relationship between premature ejaculation and chronic prostatitis/chronic pelvic pain syndrome. *The Journal of Sexual Medicine*, 12(3), 697-704.

Tran, C.N., Shoskes, D.A. (2013). Sexual dysfunction in chronic prostatitis/chronic pelvic pain syndrome. *World Journal of Urology*, 31(4), 741-6.

Chen, X., Zhou, Z., Qui, X., Wang, B., Dai, J. (2015). The effect of chronic prostatitis/chronic pelvic pain syndrome (CP/CPPS) on erectile function: a systematic review and meta-analysis. *PLOS ONE*, 10(10),e0141447. doi:10.1371/journal.pone.0141447.

Merken, H.M., Beecher, G.R. (2000). Measurement of food flavonoids by High-Performance Liquid Chromatography. *Journal of Agricultural Food Chemistry*, 48(3),577-599.

Ahluwalia, N., Andreeva, V.A., Kesse-Guyot, E., Hercberg, S. (2011). Dietary patterns, inflammation, and the metabolic syndrome. *Diabetes & Metabolism*, 39, 99-110.

Herati, A.S., Shorter, B., Srinivasan, A.K., Tai, J., Seideman, C., Lesser, M., Moldwin, R.M. (2013) Effects of foods and beverages on the symptoms of chronic prostatitis/chronic pelvic pain syndrome. *Urology*, 82(6), 1376-1380.

Aeberli, I., Gerber P.A., Hochuli, M., Kohler, S., Haile, S.R., Gouni-Berthold, I., Berthold, H.K., Spinas, G.A., & Berneis, K. (2011). Low to moderate sugar-sweetened beverage consumption impairs glucose and lipid metabolism and promotes inflammation in healthy young men: a randomized controlled trial. *The American Journal of Clinical Nutrition*, 94, 479-85.

Xiao, X., Wang, X., Gui, X, Chen, L., & Huang, B. (2016). Natural flavonoids as promising analgesic candidates: a systematic review. *Chemistry & Biodiversity*. doi: 10.1002/cbdv.201600060.

Lenoir, M., Serre, F., Cantin, L., & Ahmed, S.H.(2007). Intense sweetness surpasses cocaine reward. *PLOS ONE*, 2(8). doi:10.1371/journal.pone.0000698.

Barassi, A., Pezzilli, R., Colpi, G.M.M., Corsi, M.M., Romanelli, C., & Melzi d'Eril, G.V. (2014). Vitamin D and erectile dysfunction. *The Journal of Sexual Medicine*, 11(11), 2792-800. doi: 10.1111/jsm.12661.

Shoskes, D.A., Wang, H., Polackwich, A.S., Tucky, B., Altemus, J., & Eng, C. (2016). Analysis of gut microbiome reveals significant differences between men with chronic prostatitis/chronic pelvic pain syndrome and controls. *The Journal of Urology*, 196(2), 435-41. doi: 10.1016/j.juro.2016.02.2959.

Gallo, L. (2014). Effectiveness of diet, sexual habits and lifestyle modifications on treatment of chronic pelvic pain syndrome. *Prostate Cancer and Prostatic Disease*, 17, 238-245. doi: 10.1038/pcan.2014.18.

Carabotti, M., Scirocco, A., Maselli, M.A., & Severi, C. (2015). The gut-brain axis: interactions between enteric microbiota and central and enteric nervous system. *Annals of Gastroenterology*, 28, 203-209.

Terrier, J., & Isidori, A.M. (2016). How food intakes modify testosterone levels. *The Journal of Sexual Medicine*, 13, 1292-1296.

Sesti, F., Capozzolo, T., Pietropolli, A., Collalti, M., Bollea, M.R., & Piccione, E. (2011). Dietary therapy: a new strategy for management of chronic pelvic pain. *Nutrition Research Reviews*, 24, 31-38.

Lia, C., Lin, H., & Huang, C. (2016). Chronic prostatitis/chronic pelvic pain syndrome is associated with irritable bowel syndrome: a population-based study. *Scientific Reports*, 26, 6:26939. doi: 10.1038/srep26939.

Davidson, R.J., Kabat-Zinn, J., Schumacher, J., Rosenkranz, M., Muller, D., Santorelli, S.F., Urbanowski, F., Harrington, A., Bonus, K., & Sheridan, J.F. (2003). Alterations in brain and immune function produced by mindfulness meditation. *Psychosomatic Medicine*, 65, 564-570.

Lundh, D., Hedelin, H., Jonsson, K., Gifford, M., & Larsson, D. (2013). Assessing chronic pelvic pain syndrome, patients' blood plasma factors and cortisol saliva. *Scandinavian Journal of Urology*, 1-8.

Murphy, S.F., Schaeffer, A.J., & Thumbikat, P. (2014). Immune mediators of chronic pelvic pain syndrome: *Nature Reviews Urology*, 11(5), 259-2669. Doi:10.1038/nrurol.2014.63.

Im, H., Kim, Y., Kim H., Kim, H.S., & Son, C. (2015). Kouksundo, a traditional Korean mind-body practice, regulates oxidative stress profiles and stress hormones. *Physiology & Behavior*, 141, 9-16.

Fjorback, L.O. (2012). Mindfulness and Bodily Distress. *Danish Medical Journal*, 59(11), B4547.

Pierce, A.N., & Christianson, J.A. (2015). Stress and chronic pelvic pain. *Progress in Molecular Biology and Translational Science*, 131, 509-35. doi:10.1016/bs.pmbts.2014.11.009.

Kirby, E, D., Geraghty, A.C., Takayoshi, U., Bentley, G.E., & Kaufer, D. (2009). Stress increases putative gonadotropin inhibitory hormone and decreases luteinizing hormone in male rats. *PNAS*, 106(27), 11324-11329.

McNulty, W.H., Gevirtz, R.N., Hubbard, D.R., & Berkoff, G.M. (1994). Needle electromyographic evaluation of trigger point response to psychological stressor. *Psychophysiology*, 31, 313-316.

Kelly, D.M., & Jones, H.T. (2013). Testosterone: a vascular hormone in health and disease. *Journal of Endocrinology*, 217, R47-R71. doi: 10.1530/JOE-12-0582.

Lee, J.H. &, L. S.W. (2016). Testosterone and chronic prostatitis/chronic pelvic pain syndrome: A propensity score-matched analysis. *The Journal of Sexual Medicine*, 13(7), 1047-1055.

Louie, L. (2014). The effectiveness of yoga for depression: A critical literature review. *Issues in Mental Health Nursing*, 35, 265-276. doi: 10.3109/01612840.2013.874062.

Dhikav, V., Karmarkar, G., Verma, M., Gupta, R., Gupta, S., Mittal, D., & Anand, K. (2010). Yoga in male sexual functioning: a noncomparative pilot study. *The Journal of Sexual Medicine*, 7, 3460-3466.

Sutar, R., Yadav, S., & Desai, G. (2016). Yoga intervention and functional pain syndromes: a selective review. *International Review of Psychiatry*, 28(3), 316-22 doi: 10.1080/09540261.2016.1191448.

Field, T. (2016). Yoga research review. *Complementary Therapies in Clinical Practice*, 24, 145-161.

SpectraCell Laboratories. (2013). *Nutrient Correlation Wheels: Deficiencies Correlated with Disease Conditions*. [Booklet].

Zhang, R., Chomistek, A.K., Dimitrakoff, J.D., Giovannucci, E.L., Willett, W.C., Rosner, B.A., & Wu, K. (2015). Physical activity and chronic prostatitis/chronic pelvic pain syndrome. *Medicine & Science in Sports Exercise*. 47(4), 757-764.

Siversten, B., Lallukka, T., Petrie, K.J., Steingrimsdottir, O.A., Stubhaug. A., & Nielsen, C.S. (2015). Sleep and pain sensitivity in adults. *Pain*, 156(8), 1433-1439.

Klingler, W., Velders M., Hoppe, K., Pedro, M., & Schlep, R. (2014). Clinical relevance of fascial tissue and dysfunction. *Current Pain and Headache Reports*, 18(8), 439. doi:10.1007/s11916-014-0439-y.

Davies, C., Davies, A. (2013). *The Trigger Point Therapy Workbook. Your self-treatment guide for pain relief.* Oakland, CA: New Harbinger Publications, Inc.

Dunn, J. (2016). Save yourself from stress. *TIME Special Edition*, 17-23.

Hauser, B. (2016). Get in the sleep zone. *TIME Special Edition*, 24-27.

Rankin, L. (2016). Can you think yourself well? *TIME Special Edition*, 30-33.

Williams, M.E. (2016). Why every mind needs mindfulness. *TIME Special Edition*, 9-15.

Stedronsky, J., Pardy, B. (2006). *Myofascial Stretching: A Guide to Self-treatment*. Greenwood Village, CO: ECKO House Publishing.

Ingraham, P., & Taylor, T. (2016). Trigger Points & Myofascial Pain Syndrome: A guide to the unfinished science of muscle pain, with reviews of every theory and self-treatment and therapy option. Vancouver, CA: Paul, Ingraham (ebook tutorial).

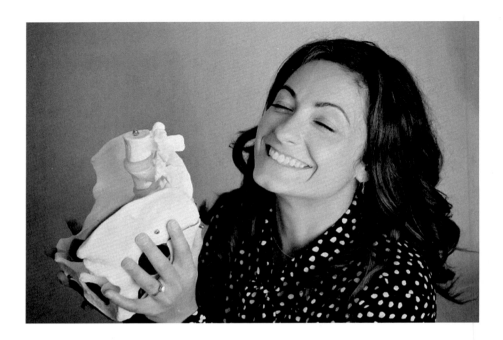

Dr. Susie Gronski is a doctor of physical therapy and a board certified pelvic rehabilitation practitioner. In addition to knowing a lot about your private parts, she's also a certified health coach.

Her passion is to make you feel comfortable about taboo subjects like sex and private parts. Social stigmas aren't her thing. She provides real advice without the medical fluff, sorta' like a friend who knows the lowdown down below.

Dr. Susie is an author and the creator of a unique hands-on training program (drsusieg.com/hands-on-training-program) helping men with pelvic pain become experts in treating themselves.

She's determined to make sure you know you can get help for:

- painful ejaculation
- problems with the joystick
- discomfort or pain during sex
- controlling your pee

without needing to be embarrassed…

So whatever you want to call it, (penis, shlong or ding-dong), if you've got a problem 'down there', she's the person to get to know. Dr. Susie is currently in private practice in Asheville, North Carolina specializing in holistic men's pelvic health. Learn more by visiting drsusieg.com.

Made in the USA
Middletown, DE
10 January 2019